CPAP is Sexy
Get Lasting Vigor & Vitality from Your CPAP

YATIN J. PATEL MD MBA FCCP

Pulmonary & Sleep Physician

ISBN-13: 978-1490947013
ISBN-10: 1490947019

DEDICATION

To my patients, especially those who hate CPAP because
they make me a better physician and a better person

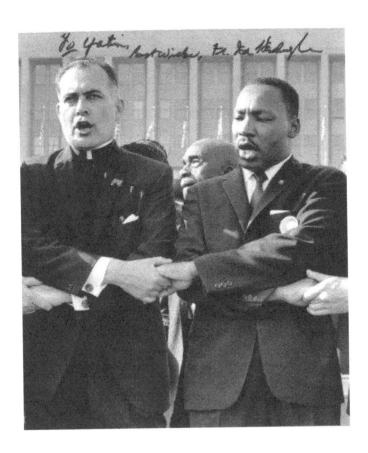

Late Father Ted Hesburgh, whose blessings made this
book possible

ACKNOWLEDGEMENT

I thank my medical assistants, Connie Schmuck, Dawn Hively, Misty Reynolds, Jennie Lynch, Tammi Gard, Pam Miller, and others, for sharing the tips and techniques with me so that I can pass those on to make your CPAP experience pleasant and rewarding.

I am also grateful to the rest of our Dream Team, Norma Coronado-Ortiz, Angie Drummond, Brenda K. Bontrager, Michelle Mishler, Kim Devine, Tiffany Lambert, Angelica Ann Adamson, Amanda Summers, Randy Perry, Tonika Hively, and Abbee Schmuck for running our clinic so smoothly that I can serve thousands of patients, and still have time to write this book.

Debbie Ponce, our nurse practitioner, made it possible for me to write this book by happily sharing the load of running our busy clinic.

Without my wife Dipti's support, this book would have taken twice as long, although sometimes, I feel that it would have taken half as long without her honey-do-lists. Nonetheless, in the spirit of world peace, I thank her for her unconditional love.

My daughters, Priyata, Pooja, and my son, Parth, politely refuse to read my books. This refusal nudges me to write more and more hoping that one day they will pick up my book and pretend to read it. I thank them for that inadvertent encouragement.

I remember my father, back home in India in the sixties and seventies, tirelessly writing and rewriting his long novels with pen and paper. This memory stimulates me to keep on typing without whining.

Lastly, I thank Lord Ganesha, who transcribed the oldest and longest epic, Mahabharata, at an unprecedented speed. Without his divine inspiration, my lazy fingers would have given up a long time ago.

The CPAP is the only intervention in the world that improves a person's physical health, attention, memory, intellectual capacity, intimacy, emotions, longevity, and thereby personal, professional, and family life.

PROLOGUE

"I don't have any sleep problem. I sleep just fine. My wife forced me to come here," a stocky engineer in his forties vented out his irritation.

"Your wife reports that you snore loudly and stop breathing all night long. You fall asleep in the recliner. You are always tired and sleepy. She is worried that you may not wake up at all."

I also explained to him that the treatment of sleep apnea reduces the risk of stroke, heart attack, high blood pressure, irregular heart rate, diabetes, dementia, drowsy driving, and early death.

Now, he got even more irritated, "I am not going to wear that thing," referring to the Continuous Positive Airway Pressure machine that the patients with sleep apnea wear during sleep to keep the airway open.

Having heard this argument often, I politely continued, "Studies have shown that the CPAP also improves intimacy, desire, and sexual function." He became quiet; his eyes slowly became big, he straightened up in the chair, trying to hide his excitement, he uttered, "Hmm... perhaps I can give it a try. How soon can I get that machine, Doc?"

Over the years, I have seen a wide variation of such responses. I am always amazed that the fear of death does not convince people to try CPAP, but that of the erectile dysfunction promptly does.

The studies indeed have shown that up to 68% of men with Obstructive Sleep Apnea report sexual dysfunction and loss of interest in sex.

In a study published in Journal of Clinical Sleep Medicine, Judith L. Reishtein, Ph.D., and colleagues evaluated the sexual function of 176 patients with sleep apnea before and after the treatment with CPAP for three months.

Intimate and sexual relationships were assessed using the Intimate and Sexual Relationships Questionnaire. This disease-specific, self-administered instrument contained 30 questions and five stand-alone subscales.

The study showed that the difficulty with sexual desire went down from 69% to 40%, arousal problems went down from 46% to 2%, and orgasm difficulties decreased from 29% to 18% after just three months of treatment with CPAP.

Those who are sleepier, as the researcher found, may be less interested and more impaired in sexual activity. Indeed, Barnes and colleagues also found among a group of 98 men with OSA, those with Erectile Dysfunction were significantly sleepier in the daytime than those without ED. Frequent apnea episodes rob you of your stage 3 and stage REM (Rapid Eye Movement) sleep making you wake up sleepy. This morning tiredness, according to the study by Margel and colleagues, is predictive of sexual dissatisfaction and the inability to have a morning erection.

In addition to excessive sleepiness, other potential mechanisms have been considered, including low testosterone levels as well as the lack of oxygen causing the dysfunction of the nerves responsible for erection.

"My doctors are puzzled as to why my testosterone level is zero. It is not low; it is zero. My doctor has never seen zero testosterone. I have seen three different endocrinologists, who have done a thorough work-up and have not been able to find a cause of this," a frustrated young man with moderately severe sleep apnea shared with me. I reassured him that there is a good chance that the CPAP treatment will improve his testosterone level.

In a study of 1312 men, Barrett-Connor and colleagues found that men with the lowest testosterone levels had more severe apnea than those with normal levels. They also spent more of their sleep time with oxygen saturation less than 90%.

Soukhova-O'Hare found that the chronic intermittent hypoxemia (lack of oxygen caused by sleep apnea) produced a 55% decrease in the number of daily spontaneous erections that were reversed after six weeks of recovery from hypoxemia. They also found reduced sexual drive and mating activity.

Thus, the findings from these studies suggest that the effect of OSA on intimate and sexual behaviors may be multifactorial, but the good news is that the treatment with CPAP restores sexual function within several weeks.

Bradshaw and colleagues demonstrated a significant increase in the Intimate and Sexual Relationships score in participants who received just two weeks of CPAP treatment.

Goncalves and colleagues reported Erectile Dysfunction resolved in 13 of 17 OSA patients treated for one month with CPAP.

Akashiba and colleagues reported that in patients with severe OSA, following six weeks CPAP treatment, Intimacy and Sexual Relationships scores improved significantly.

The treatment of sleep apnea with CPAP improves intimacy and sexual function in both men and women. The research has not yet focused on women's sexual dysfunction, but my experience has been similar in both sexes. My female patients with sleep apnea have complained of the lack of desire and interest in sex. Some of them have reported difficulty with orgasm. These symptoms improve promptly with CPAP treatment. Additionally, besides enhancing the love for your partner, this treatment will also restore the love for your work, and for your life.

It will also reduce your risk of stroke, heart attack, high blood pressure, abnormalities of heart rhythm, congestive heart failure, high blood sugar, seizures, rheumatoid arthritis, acid reflux, asthma exacerbations, and drowsy driving. So, listen to your spouse and talk to us.

In the following pages, I have tried to convince you to get diagnosed and treated for sleep apnea.

I understand that sleeping with CPAP is an adjustment, a huge lifestyle change, and for some, akin to sleeping with an enemy, but it is worth it. I have tons of patients, who were reluctant to start this therapy, but now they would not even nap without a CPAP. They have experienced first-hand the improvement this treatment makes in their alertness, energy level, mood, personality, and health.

The studies have shown that early intensive education improves CPAP compliance. Based on the current medical evidence and my experience of working with thousands of patients over last twenty-five years, I explain why and how you should use CPAP. I also help you choose the right equipment and proper accessories to make your use as comfortable as possible.

I have seen quite a few patients who are feeling sleepy despite using CPAP every night, mainly because of poor sleep habits. The CPAP use does not improve your sleep if you drink caffeine all day, use alcohol within 3-4 hours of bedtime, worry about your problems while in bed, and maintain an irregular sleep-wakefulness schedule.

Hence, I have emphasized how you can be maximally alert all-day long using sleep hygiene. You can leverage your alertness to get the most out of your life by learning the revolutionary tool called AEI Model of Supreme Life. This model teaches you how to squeeze out maximum life from each moment by managing your Alertness, Emotions, and Intelligence.

This book is divided into the following five sections:

Section I:
Sleep? Who Cares?
What Is Sleep Apnea?

This section describes sleep physiology, including various sleep stages, their functions, and, most interestingly, the rapid eye movement (REM) sleep.

What is micro-sleep?
How much sleep do I need?
Can I sleep less and live more?

Describes Obstructive Sleep Apnea - its symptoms, its diagnosis with a convenient home sleep test, and the consequences of untreated sleep apnea.

Who should be tested for sleep apnea?
What are the symptoms?
Do I have to go to the sleep lab?
What are the limitations of the home sleep test?

Section II
Why You Should Use CPAP

This section gives you the medical studies proving the dangers of untreated sleep apnea and the benefits of CPAP treatment; Congestive Heart Failure, irregular heart rhythm, uncontrolled blood pressure, diabetes, kidney disease, seizure disorder, depression, attention deficit hyperactivity, rheumatoid arthritis, drowsy driving, fibromyalgia, weight gain, pregnancy, and cancer.

It then explains the comprehensive benefits of the treatment to your health, alertness, personality, mood, and executive function.

Section III
How You Should Use CPAP

This section gives you the evidence-based and experience-based answers to the common problems you may encounter.

It describes various treatment options including CPAP, oral appliance, and hypoglossal nerve stimulation.

It answers the following questions:

Which machine and interface should I use?
Should I buy a travel CPAP?
Will my insurance cover the cost?
I have a high-deductible insurance. How can I get treated with least amount of money?

What are the advantages of a humidifier?
I hate the big, bulky, monstrous masks. What can I do?
Will the noise keep my spouse awake?
I toss and turn all-night. Can I still use CPAP?
I suffer from claustrophobia. What should I do?
I sleep with my face buried in a pillow.
I drool in the mask.
I wake up with a dry mouth.

This section also provides tips to help CPAP-users during menstruation, pregnancy, and menopause.

There are tips to help insomnia patients sleep well with CPAP.

Section IV
Sound Sleep Habits Lead to an Alert Life

The CPAP use does not protect you from poor habits that can rob you of your deep stages of sleep and thereby of your life.

This section describes good sleep habits that will give you the most restorative sleep and earn you the most return on your investment in sleep

It arms you with the tips to help you achieve rectangular alertness—maximal alertness that can last all day long.

This section also teaches you the technique of power nap - Patel's Relaxed Eye Muscles (PREM) nap, a revolutionary power-nap technique that can restore alertness and excellence despite sleep debt

Once I start using CPAP, can I get by with just 4 hours of sleep?

This section focuses on sleep debt and its ill effects on alertness, emotional intelligence, informational intelligence, and, thereby, executive performance.

Section V
Live a Supreme Life on CPAP

This section incorporates all we have learned into an integrative model; the AEI Model of Supreme Life. This revolutionary model teaches you to get the most life out of your sleep by starting with CPAP use, and then adding good sleep habits, and then ultimately learning to manage Alertness, Emotions, and Information even when faced with crises.

It teaches how to leverage alertness to achieve maximal emotional intelligence and informational intelligence and to reach AEImax, a state of consistent excellence

It takes the concept even further by adding selflessness and spiritual force to achieve AEI∞.

Sleep Deeply. Live Fully. Love Truly.

Treat your sleep disorder with discipline. Then protect your sleep, both in duration and in quality, with the same tenacity you guard your life as both are intricately tied together.

Remember that we are here on this beautiful earth for only a finite amount of time. The only way we can squeeze maximum life out of each moment is by maximizing our alertness, even during stressful periods. It is an uphill battle, but with patience, perseverance, practice, and faith, you shall excel and enjoy despite unavoidable sleep debt.

Guard your sleep like you guard your life. And when you cannot get sufficient sleep because of stress at home or at work, use the LAMP (Leader's Alertness Maximization Plan) to maximize alertness. Leverage this alertness to maximize your emotional intelligence and informational intelligence. Add selflessness and spirituality to this mix, and you will maximize your God-given potential.

Section I

Sleep? Who Cares?
Why Treat Sleep Apnea?

Whose woods these are I think I know.
His house is in the village, though;
He will not see me stopping here
To watch his woods fill up with snow.

My little horse must think it queer
To stop without a farmhouse near
Between the woods and frozen lake
The darkest evening of the year.

He gives his harness bells a shake
To ask if there is some mistake.
The only other sounds the sweep
Of easy wind and downy flake.

The woods are lovely, dark, and deep,
But I have promises to keep,
And miles to go before I sleep,
And miles to go before I sleep.

- Robert Frost

Normal Sleep

In this age of abundant opportunity for advancement and entertainment, we too have miles to go before we sleep. This is the reason some of us look at sleep as an enemy of life; something that prevents us from getting things done. Nothing could be farther from truth. Sound sleep, in fact, allows us to live and work better, and for a longer period. It also makes us happier, smarter, and healthier.

Until the 1950s, most people thought of sleep as a passive, dormant part of our daily lives. Sleep, in fact, is an active and organized process.

Nerve-signaling chemicals called neurotransmitters control whether we are asleep or awake by acting on different groups of nerve cells, or neurons, in the brain. Neurons in the brainstem, which connects the brain with the spinal cord, produce neurotransmitters such as serotonin and norepinephrine that keep some parts of the brain active while we are awake. Other neurons at the base of the brain begin signaling when we fall asleep. These neurons appear to "switch off" the signals that keep us awake. Research also suggests that a chemical called adenosine builds up in our blood while we are awake and causes drowsiness. This chemical gradually breaks down while we sleep.

The sleep state includes two major types of sleep: REM (Rapid Eye Movements) sleep and non-REM (NREM) sleep. NREM sleep is divided into three different stages, with stage three referred to as "delta sleep." In adults, NREM sleep accounts for approximately 80 percent of their sleeping time, while REM sleep occupies 20 percent of the normal sleep experience.

Our sleep consists of sleep cycles of about ninety minutes each, during which we cycle through light (NREM stage 1 and 2) sleep and deep (NREM stage 3, and REM) sleep. On a typical night, we go through four to five such cycles, and with each cycle, our REM sleep gets longer, deeper, and more restorative.

The REM sleep paradoxically is the active most state of our existence with vivid dreams tracked continually by darting eyes. It is characterized by intense activity in the cerebral hemisphere contrasting with a total paralysis of all the skeletal muscles except the diaphragm and the eye muscles. This paralysis prevents us from acting out our dreams. Interestingly, penile tumescence (clitoral erection and vaginal engorgement) occur during REM sleep. This fact can help men differentiate between psychogenic and organic impotence. If you wake up with an erection, you do not have organic impotence.

Sleep helps your brain work properly. While we are sleeping, our brain is preparing for the next day. It's forming new pathways to help us learn and remember information.

Studies show that a good night's sleep improves learning. Whether we are learning math, how to play the piano, how to perfect golf swing, or how to drive a car, sleep helps enhance our learning and problem-solving skills.

It plays a vital role in memory consolidation, information processing, and retrieval. Adequate duration of regular sleep is necessary to maintain normal levels of cognitive skills such as memory, speech, complex thinking, and creative problem-solving.

Sleep helps maintain a healthy balance of the hormones that make you feel hungry (ghrelin) or full (leptin). When we don't get enough sleep, our level of ghrelin goes up, and the level of leptin goes down. This makes us feel hungrier than usual.

Sleep also affects how our body reacts to insulin, the hormone that controls our blood glucose (sugar) level. Sleep deficiency results in a higher than normal blood sugar level, which may increase our risk for diabetes.

Our immune system relies on sleep to stay healthy. This system defends our body against foreign or harmful substances. Ongoing sleep deficiency can change the way in which your immune system responds. For example, if sleep deficient, we may have trouble fighting common infections.

Lack of sleep also may lead to micro-sleep. Micro-sleep refers to brief moments of sleep that occur when you're normally awake.

You cannot control micro-sleep, and you might not be aware of it. For example, have you ever driven somewhere and then not remembered part of the trip? If so, you may have experienced micro-sleep.

Even if you're not driving, micro-sleep can affect how you function. If you're listening to a lecture, for example, you might miss some of the information or feel like you don't understand the point. In reality, though, you may have slept through part of the lecture and not been aware of it. You, just now, might have experienced micro-sleep while reading about micro-sleep!

Some people aren't aware of the risks of sleep deficiency. In fact, they may not even realize that they are sleep deficient. Even with limited or poor-quality sleep, they may still think that they can function well.

For example, drowsy drivers may feel capable of driving. Yet, studies show that sleep deficiency harms your driving ability as much as, or more than, being drunk. It's estimated that driver sleepiness is a factor in about 100,000 car accidents each year, resulting in about 1,500 deaths.

Drivers are not the only ones affected by sleep deficiency. It can affect people in all lines of work, including health care workers, pilots, students, lawyers, mechanics, and assembly line workers.

As a result, sleep deficiency is not only harmful on a personal level, but it also can cause large-scale damage. For example, sleep deficiency has played a role in human errors linked to tragic accidents, such as nuclear reactor meltdowns, grounding of large ships, and aviation accidents.

The patients with untreated sleep apnea often tell me that they sleep just fine. What they do not realize is that they are spending more time in the lighter (NREM 1 and 2) stages of sleep at the expense of the deeper (NREM 3 and REM) stages of sleep. This distortion of the sleep architecture impairs the function of the prefrontal cortex, an area in the front of our brain that is necessary for accurate self-assessment. Once they get on CPAP, do they realize how sleepy, tired, and grumpy they were.

How Much Sleep Do I need?

This is the commonest question I get asked when I give talks about sleep. "Whatever it takes for you to feel maximally alert all-day, from the time you wake up to the time you go back to bed!" is what I tell them. Most adults need 7 to 8 hours of sleep to feel alert and energetic. This sleep need is as unique as your fingerprint, though. For you, it can be 7 hours, for your spouse, it can be 8 hours, and for your best friend, it may only be 6 and a half hours.

Until recently we did not have a clear-cut, evidence-based recommendation as to the duration of sleep needed for a healthy life. But, in June 2015, a panel of 15 experts from the American Academy of Sleep Medicine and the Sleep Research Society, after reviewing 5314 scientific articles, concluded that adults need 7 or more hours of sleep every night.

Here, are their specific recommendations:

1. Sleeping less than 7 hours per night is associated with adverse health outcomes, including weight gain, diabetes, hypertension, heart disease, stroke, depression, and increased risk of death. It is also associated with impaired immune function, increased pain, poor performance, increased errors, and greater risk of accidents.

2. Sleeping more than 9 hours per night on a regular basis may be appropriate for young adults, individuals recovering from sleep debt, and individuals with illnesses. For others, it is uncertain whether sleeping more than 9 hours per night is associated with health risk.

3. People concerned they are sleeping too little or too much should consult their healthcare provider.

Please note that above recommendations do answer that question our overworking adults ask: "Can I earn more money if I sleep less? Can I get more life if I sleep less?" It is a legitimate question, and the answer is, "No, you cannot. Not for long."

Dr. Van Dongen and colleagues at the University of Pennsylvania studied participants after four, six, and eight hours of sleep for fourteen days and found a significant dose-dependent decline in their neurological and cognitive performance. Thus, by sleeping less, you can read more, but you will remember less. You can check more e-mails, but your responses will not reflect your true leadership skills. You can interact with more people, but you will be less perceptive. You can work on more problems, but your solutions will be less creative. In short, if you are sleeping less, you might be a liability, as opposed to an asset.

By sleeping less, you are not only increasing your risk of diseases mentioned above but also impairing your executive function — creativity, problem-solving, communication, and goal-directed behavior. These are the reasons why business giants like Warren Buffet, Bill Gates, and Satya Nadela try to get 7-8 hours sleep despite their busy schedules.

Bill Gates gets at least seven hours of sleep a night because "that's what I need to stay sharp and creative and upbeat." Jeff Bezos, CEO of Amazon.com, says, "I'm more alert, and I think more clearly if I've had eight hours' sleep."

What about Indira Gandhi, Margaret Thatcher, Indra Nooyi of Pepsi and the likes, who claimed to sleep only 4-5 hours a night? Could they need less sleep? Do they carry a short-sleeper gene? Well, Dr. Ying-Hui Fu and at his team at the University of California, San Francisco, did find that short-sleeper gene, a rare mutation, but it is present in only 3 percent of the population. Dr. Ying-Hui Fu himself commented that while these people sleep less than 6 hours, but he does not know if they are at an increased risk for various diseases because of their short sleep.

My overworked colleagues, unaware of the research cited above, continue to argue against sufficient sleep. Here is a list of arguments made by these skeptics and my responses:

1. *I don't need eight hours of sleep.*
   Studies have shown that restricting sleep to four or six hours (compared to eight hours) for fourteen days causes a dose-dependent decline in your executive function.

2. *I only need five hours of sleep.*
   The short-sleeper gene, a rare mutation, is present in only 3 percent of the population (Ying-Hui Fu, University of California, San Francisco). The majority of the working people worldwide get less than six hours of sleep, certainly during a major opportunity or catastrophe.

3. *I can fight sleep deprivation with strong motivation.*
   Motivation improves attention but not creativity, flexibility, mood, perception, and information management.

4. *I have achieved a lot by sleeping less.*
   You could achieve even more by sleeping more.

5. *I don't perceive the deficit in my performance.*
   Sleep deprivation adversely affects prefrontal cortex (area of

the brain called "the executive center"), which is essential for successful self-evaluation. This makes us unaware of our deficit.

6. *I am highly productive.* You have increased your output as a worker, at the expense of leadership output. You are compromising the quality at the expense of quantity.

7. *I don't want to sleep away a third of my life.* Investment in sleep will enrich your life qualitatively, both at home and at work.

I have made my case for 7-8 hours of sleep every night, but what if you are feeling sleepy and tired despite sleeping 8 hours every night?

First make sure you are getting quality sleep by following good sleep habits; keeping a regular sleep schedule even on weekends, exercising 30 minutes a day, not working in bed, avoiding caffeine after 1 PM, not eating a large meal before bedtime, not consuming alcohol within 3 hours of bedtime and most importantly, praying before retiring to sleep. Then, make sure you do not suffer from depression or Obstructive Sleep Apnea - a disease characterized by loud snoring and cessation of breathing for 10 or more seconds all night long.

In conclusion, invest richly in sleep and get the most out of your limited stay on this beautiful earth. Make a commitment, as a family, to get 7-8 hours of sound sleep every night. Enjoy lasting alertness, energy, vigor, and vitality; and live a healthy, happy, and a long life.

I will leave you with a favorite shloka of mine. (Bhagavad Gita,

Chapter 6:17)

> yuktahara-viharasya yukta-cestasya karmasu,
> yukta-svapnavabodhasya, yogo bhavati duhkha-ha.

A person who is temperate in eating, sleeping, working, and recreation can mitigate all material pains by practicing the yoga system.

What is Obstructive Sleep Apnea?

Obstructive sleep apnea, a serious and potentially fatal disorder, affects approximately twenty-six percent of the male and nine percent of females between 30 - 60 years of age. It is much more common in males, but after menopause, this gap narrows as the hormonal changes make females' upper airway more collapsible.

When we started our sleep center in 1994, the consensus was that sleep apnea is a disease of heavy men. But now we are finding more and more females, and thin patients with sleep apnea, because fat deposition around the airway is only one of the risk factors for this disease. There are genetic, familial, and anatomic factors that can cause repeated collapse of the upper airway.

Snoring, daytime fatigue, witnessed apnea (cessation of respiration for more than ten-seconds sometimes as long as a minute), morning headaches, dry throat, and waking up gasping for air are common features of this disorder, which is being increasingly recognized as a formidable enemy of life. There are also patients, even with severe apnea, who will deny symptoms. "I sleep fine. I don't have a problem with daytime sleepiness." Only after the CPAP treatment, do they realize how sleepy and tired they were.

Sleep apnea prevents a person from reaching deep, restorative stages of sleep, making the person grumpy, irritable, nervous, forgetful, inattentive, and tired. It also increases the risk of stroke, heart attack, and early death because of the nightly struggle to breathe, which causes frequent elevation of blood pressure and sustained drop in blood oxygen level, while simultaneously increasing the oxygen consumption of the heart muscles. Untreated, sleep apnea increases the risk of motor vehicular and industrial accidents.

Take the STOP-BANG questionnaire to determine your risk for obstructive sleep apnea:

Do you **S**nore loudly?

Do you often feel **T**ired, fatigued, or sleepy during daytime?

Has anyone **O**bserved you stop breathing during sleep?

Do you have or are you being treated for high blood **P**ressure?

Is your **B**MI >35kg/m2?

Is your **A**ge greater than 50 years?

Is your **N**eck circumference bigger than 40 cm?

Are you male **G**ender?

Patients with three or more positive responses should get evaluated for obstructive sleep apnea.

You can also watch my 90-sec video clip from PBS to learn about the symptoms of sleep apnea https://youtu.be/bE_BUlcFm8Y.

Most patients can be diagnosed by a home sleep test, which is quick, convenient, and significantly cheaper than an in-lab sleep study. You can also watch my video about home sleep test at https://youtu.be/VYmo5LLgs30.

The graph below shows dangerous drops in the oxygen level in a young salesperson with uncontrolled blood pressure and blood sugars, elevated cholesterol, and excessive daytime sleepiness.

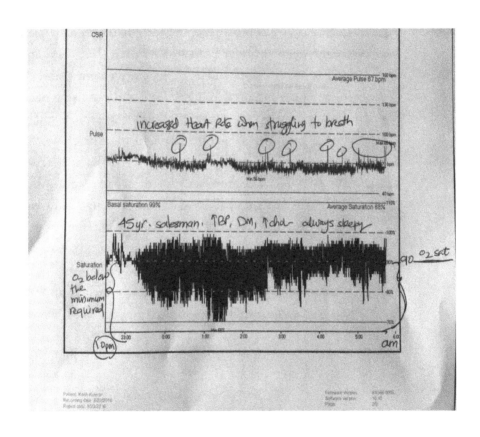

Please notice the sudden increase in the heart rate repeatedly during the night. This young man dropped off his home test device to come back several days later for the treatment discussion. Worried about his desaturations, Misty, our medical assistant, put him in the examination room right away, and asked me to see him. We got him started on the CPAP right away.

If the home sleep test is equivocal, then you may need an overnight sleep study in a sleep lab where your respirations, oxygen level, heart rate, EKG, leg movements, and sleep stages will be monitored all night long without using needles. The commonest and most successful treatment includes wearing a mask or a cannula hooked to a machine, called continuous positive airway pressure (CPAP), which acts as a pneumatic splint and prevents your throat from collapsing at night. As one of our patient, a pleasant young lady with a history depression, put it, "I can't believe something as simple as blowing air in the throat can change someone's life!"

It is extremely rewarding to be treated for sleep apnea. My patients over the years have told me:

"Doc, I did not know how sleepy I was until I started wearing CPAP."

"A hazy screen has been lifted off from my face."

"I thought it was all stress and aging, but now I feel young again."

"I am thinking clearer. I am planning better. I am getting more done at work and home."

"I have so much energy that I don't know what to do with it."

"My blood pressure is better; my sugars are better controlled."

"I should have done this a long time ago."

"For the first time in decades, I am dreaming!"

"My coworkers have noticed my energy and enthusiasm."

"My son wakes up with wide awake eyes. He comes home, and he talks to us instead of dozing off. He drove to Florida last week."

"Even though I didn't feel tired before, now I am feeling different; better, more alert!"

"I wake up before the alarm goes off. I used to have two loud alarms, and still, I will sleep through them and be late to work."

"Doc, I am dreaming deeper. Dreams are more pleasant and more vivid."

If you suspect you have sleep apnea, please talk to your doctor. It will give you a new life. If you need additional information, please read my blog at http://SnoozeClinic.com, or watch my videos on http://www.youtube.com/yjpatel.

Whenever in Doubt, Repeat the Test

This pleasant thirty year old lady with snoring, fatigue, and insomnia had a normal home sleep test, but doubted the accuracy of her normal home sleep test saying, "I did not sleep well that night." Her apnea hypopnea index was normal at 3 per hour.

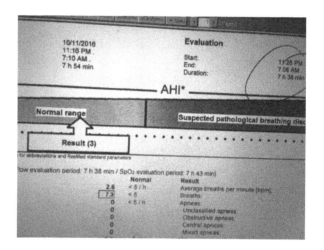

We discussed the option of repeating the home test versus dong an in-lab sleep test, which is the gold standard. We ordered an in-lab sleep study (her insurance fortunately approved it) and it did show this severe obstructive sleep apnea with apnea hypopnea index of 82 per hour as seen in the following report.

...below. This results in a normal sleep efficiency of
al. Latency to initial REM sleep is normal. During the
I sleep and slow wave sleep Very limited REM sleep
her right side. She exhibited 146 obstructive apneas
ly increased apnea/hypopnea index of 82 events per
d nonsupine. They are more frequent while in a supine
agmented sleep. They were also associated with
ded was 81%. She desaturated 3% or more below her
e night, the patient does exhibit frequent light to

We have never seen such a huge discrepancy between
the home test and in-lab test, but it can occur if the person
does not spend enough time in the deeper stages of sleep or
in supine position during the home sleep test. Remember,
the home sleep test is a screening test only. If it is equivocal,
insist on repeating it or even getting an in-lab sleep test.

I don't have a sleep problem!

I hear this all the time. Sleep apnea is a perfect disease to be in denial. You are asleep. How do you know that you snore and that you stop breathing? Such denial is the reason that the majority of sleep apnea patients go undiagnosed.

"I sleep just fine. I don't even snore. I certainly don't stop breathing. I am tired during daytime, but I am working too much and I am approaching the big 50. It is nothing unusual."

Some of you are still in denial even after the home sleep test shows sleep apnea. You just do not want to accept that you will have to change the behavior. You will have to sleep with a cannula or a mask. You assume it will be uncomfortable. You will have to wear it every night. You will have to travel with the CPAP.

The diagnosis comes as a shock to quite a few patients. Even though, I don't have sleep apnea, I can understand that shock. A couple of years ago, I was in a state of shock and disbelief when my routine blood test results came back showing diabetes. I knew that I will have diabetes sooner or later as both my parents were diagnosed with diabetes in their sixties. I was sedentary, but slim. I ate sensibly most days. I did not expect that I will be stuck with that diagnosis this soon and will have to quit eating dessert at 50! I just could not see myself pricking my fingers either multiple times a day.

I remember the day the blood test results delivered me that shocking news. The unexpected results came back on a cloudy, dreary, Friday morning in the fall as I was seeing patients in the clinic. I focused hard on the task at hand and finished my clinic work and went home.

That evening, we had a few doctor friends from the hospital over for dinner. To divert my attention from the diagnosis of diabetes, I slipped into my usual role of a self-proclaimed mixologist. I started serving drinks - Chardonnay for my wife, Malbec for Dr. Vijay Mehta, masala ginger ale for Mrs. Mehta, Mandarin Martini for Dr. Neelam Patel and his wife. For Dr. Bhagat, I made his favorite, Mint Cilantro Mojito with extra sugar per his preference. He took a sip of his Mojito, gave me an unflattering look, and right away reached for more sugar, and added a large spoon of sugar proudly saying, "My blood sugar is normal! My cholesterol is not bad either!"

As you can imagine, my mood sank deeper. Now, I can't enjoy my favorite Cadbury chocolates from England or Crème Brule from the local Corn Dance tavern, not to mention a few Indian delicacies I have been addicted to since my prior births!

It took me a month to adjust to this new reality. I had to convince myself that my body cannot digest sugar. It is a poison for me. I remember Mahatma Gandhi's quote - Renunciation without Repugnance is a Torture. Hence, I started developing an intense dislike towards everything sweet. I practiced saying, "I don't like sweets. My body can't handle sugar." As a result, I, not only quit sweet, but also minimized carbs. I also picked up swimming and bike riding as running was hurting my knee cap. Two months' later, my sugars were normal without any medications. And more importantly, I feel more energetic, alert, and healthy. I have never felt this good ever in my life; during my childhood, I was always sick because of my allergies and asthma.

You can do this too. You can adjust to sleeping with CPAP. You can turn the whole ordeal into a nightly routine. It may not be easy, but it will be well worth the effort. CPAP will give you your life back. It will improve your health. It will infuse more love in your family life. It will energize your professional life. And all these would happen as soon as you start using your CPAP. I see such miracles every day.

You can use similar resolve for weight loss, which in case of mild apnea, may cure you of your sleep apnea besides providing other health benefits.

In the following section, you can read about the medical studies proving the benefits of CPAP use. You know that the CPAP is beneficial for you and your health, but reading these studies will provide you an insight into these wide-ranging benefits. It will solidify your resolve and improve your compliance.

Section II
Why You Should Use CPAP

"Do you enjoy this?" a sixty-six-year-old lady, who volunteers at the Habitat for Humanity asked me with a smile referring to my sleep medicine practice, as I was explaining her the home sleep test procedure.

"Love it infinity times infinity," as my kids used to say!

"There is nothing else in the world that can improve a person's health, longevity, mood, energy level, and executive function to this degree and this quickly. Something as simple as blowing a little air in your throat can transform your personal, professional, and family life in just one night! I am honored that I can play a small part in that metamorphosis every single day. Mine is the most gratifying life one can hope to lead."

Sleep Apnea increases Long-term Complications after Bypass Surgery

Obstructive Sleep Apnea is independently associated with a higher rate of long-term cardiovascular events after Coronary Artery Bypass Graft surgery (CABG).

Sixty-seven consecutive patients referred for CABG underwent clinical evaluation and standard sleep study in the preoperative period. The primary end point was Major Adverse Cardiac or Cerebrovascular Events (MACCEs) (combined events of all-cause death, heart attack, repeated angioplasty[1], and stroke). Secondary end points included individual MACCEs, typical angina pain, and heart rhythm disturbances. Patients were evaluated at 30 days (short-term) and up to 6.1 years (long term) after CABG.

---

[1] Opening blocked arteries during heart catheterization using a balloon

OSA (apnea-hypopnea index $\geq$ 15 events/h) was present in 56% of the population. The patients were followed for a mean of 4.5 years (range, 3.2-6.1 years).

In contrast, MACCE (35% vs 16%), new angioplasty or stent placement (19% vs 0%), episodes of typical angina (30% vs 7%), and atrial fibrillation[2] (22% vs 0%) were more common in patients with than without OSA in the long-term follow-up.

OSA was an independent factor associated with the occurrence of MACCE, repeated angioplasty, typical angina, and atrial fibrillation in the multivariate analysis. So, if you or your loved one has gone through bypass surgery, please get tested and treated for sleep apnea. This will reduce the risk of death, heart attack, stroke, and irregular heart rate.CPAP Reduces the Risk of Repeat Angioplasty

Between 2002 and 2012, Xiaofan Wu, MD, and colleagues identified 390 patients with OSA who had undergone angioplasty of the blocked coronary arteries. Obstructive Sleep Apnea was diagnosed in these patients through in-laboratory sleep studies and defined by an apnea-hypopnea (apnea = cessation of respirations, hypopnea = abnormally shallow respiration for longer than 10 seconds) index $\geq$ five events/h. The median follow-up period was 4.8 years.

The untreated moderate-severe OSA group had a higher incidence of blockage of coronary artery needing a repeat angioplasty than the treated moderate-severe OSA group

---

[2] A rapid and irregular heart rhythm

(25.1% vs. 14.1%). CPAP treatment reduced this risk.

CPAP Reduces Congestive Heart Failure Exacerbations

Wearing CPAP every night can be a challenge for some, but a study published in The American Journal of Cardiology gives one more reason to be compliant with CPAP.

"The regular use of CPAP in patients, hospitalized with decompensated congestive heart failure is associated with a reduction in readmissions," said first author Sunil Sharma, M.D., FAASM, Associate Professor of Pulmonary Medicine at the Thomas Jefferson University.

Dr. Sharma and his team screened patients admitted to the hospital with heart failure, for sleep apnea. Of the seventy-five patients that followed up with an outpatient sleep study, seventy patients received the diagnosis of sleep apnea. Over the next six months, the team tracked patients' PAP compliance, emergency room visits, and readmissions. Compliance was monitored objectively by the device computer and defined as a minimum of four hours of use, 70 percent of the time, for four weeks consecutively or more during the first three months of therapy.

CPAP compliant patients had a significant reduction in readmissions for CHF.

In this study, the identification and treatment of sleep apnea in CHF patients was associated with reduced readmissions over six months after discharge. Adherence to the treatment reduced the exacerbations of Congestive Heart

Failure.

This study gives you a strong reason to wear CPAP every night, even when traveling. You do not want to wake up tired, sleepy, and short of breath.

Obstructive Sleep Apnea Worsens Heart Function Even in the Absence of Congestive Heart Failure

A study published in the Journal of Clinical Sleep Medicine indicates that Obstructive Sleep Apnea is associated with the dysfunction of the heart muscles even in the absence of Congestive Heart Failure.

A total of 79 patients with sleep apnea, but preserved systolic (squeezing) function of the heart were enrolled. Sixty-five patients were classified to have moderate to severe OSA (apnea-hypopnea index [AHI] $\geq$ 15/h), while the other 14 patients with mild or no OSA (AHI < 15/h) served as control subjects.

The researchers found that, in patients with moderate to severe OSA, the left atrium was larger, and the left ventricle was stiffer. Notably, Apnea Hypopnea Index (number of times a patient stops breathing per hour) in Rapid Eye Movement sleep was significantly correlated with the aortic root size indicating that this major blood vessel, the aorta was significantly larger in these patients.

Patients with moderate to severe OSA tend to have cardiac dysfunction revealed by echocardiography even in the absence of heart disease. High AHI in REM sleep is significantly associated with cardiac muscle remodeling and ventricular diastolic dysfunction (difficulty with relaxing and filling) and may be a potential variable to predict cardiac dysfunction.

This study gives you a valid reason to use CPAP even if you do not suffer from a heart disease.

OSA and Dangerous Heart Rhythm

OSA approximately doubles the risk of Atrial Fibrillation; an irregular and rapid rhythm that can cause palpitation, and precipitate congestive heart failure and also cause a stroke. Also, the studies of circadian rhythm and sudden cardiac death have shown that obstructive apnea may predispose an individual to sudden death in sleep.

There are multiple pathological reasons (with the subnormal levels of oxygen in the center) as described by Dr. Anna May in the January 2017 issue of the journal, Chest. In simple terms, though, just imagine someone standing next to your bed and stuffing pillow on your face all night long for ten seconds to a minute repeatedly. Imagine what this will do to your blood pressure, heart rate, and to the levels of your stress hormones.

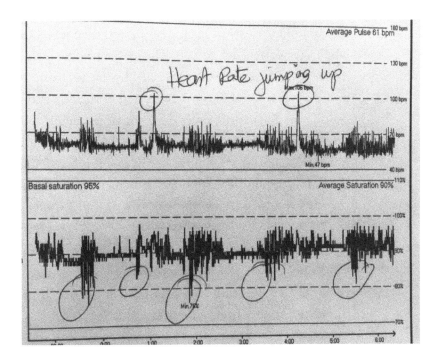

Above is the home sleep test report on a man in his forties. Note how frequently his oxygen level drops below ninety and the corresponding increase in the heart rate. This is the reason I tell my patients, especially those with moderate to severe sleep apnea that they should use CPAP even during a nap.

Quite a few patients take the CPAP off to use the restroom in the early morning hours and then leave it off when they come back to bed. The early morning is the time of deepest REM sleep characterized by the severe most drop in the oxygen level. This is when atrial fibrillation and other serious rhythm disturbances occur most frequently. Sudden deaths are also more common during the early morning hours. You also get the most rest during this REM stage sleep. Please put the CPAP back on when you wake up in the early morning hours.

Untreated sleep apnea increases your risk of recurrent atrial fibrillation and other abnormalities of heart rate and rhythm. A recent study also showed that the risk of recurrent blood clot (pulmonary embolism) in the lung is also increased in these patients. Pulmonary Embolism can be fatal if untreated.

My Blood Pressure Was High in the Morning

"My family doc told me to get checked out for sleep apnea because my blood pressure was high in the morning. I did not have any problem staying awake," a fifty-five-year-old obese male (BMI 38), a plumbing contractor, told me. His home sleep test showed a moderate sleep apnea with the apnea-hypopnea index of 21/hour. We started him on CPAP right away.

His blood pressure was 102/76 when I saw him on a Monday morning for the CPAP follow-up.

"The top number on my blood pressure used to be 200 before CPAP. I also used to wake up with a headache. The first thing I used to do every morning was to take a couple of aspirins. It did take about a couple of months for me to feel better."

"My doctor said he might take me off my Norvasc on next visit," he added happily.

To Reduce the Complications, Tell Anesthesiologist if You Snore

Dr. Abdelsattar and his colleagues at University of Michigan studied the impact of untreated Obstructive Sleep Apnea (OSA) on Cardiopulmonary Complications during surgery and published their findings in the journal SLEEP (Volume 38 Issue 08.)

Of 26,842 patients they studied, 2,646 had a diagnosis or suspicion of OSA. Of those, 1,465 (55.4%) were untreated. Compared with treated OSA, untreated OSA was independently associated with more cardiopulmonary complications (risk-adjusted rates 6.7% versus 4.0%), particularly unplanned reintubations (having to put the patient back on the respirator) and heart attack.

The researchers found that the patients with obstructive sleep apnea (OSA) who are not treated with positive airway pressure preoperatively are at increased risks for cardiopulmonary complications after general and vascular surgery. Improving the recognition of OSA and ensuring adequate treatment may be a strategy to reduce the risk for surgical patients with OSA.

OSA is increasingly being recognized as a risk factor for adverse postoperative complications. Despite the growing awareness of OSA's effect on postoperative outcomes, up to 80% of patients presenting for surgery may have undiagnosed OSA and are therefore untreated for this condition. In other words, adults may present for surgery without adequate preoperative risk assessment for OSA, possibly putting them at heightened risk for postoperative complications. Therefore, the American Society of

Anesthesiologists (ASA) has issued practice guidelines specific to the perioperative management of patients with OSA. In these guidelines, the ASA recommends screening patients for OSA before surgery and implementing special care pathways if OSA is present.

Hence, if you or a family member is planned to have a surgery, please tell your anesthesia doctor that you snore so that the team can take the necessary precautions to prevent these complications. It is even better if you tell this to your family physician a month prior the surgery so that the diagnosis and treatment of sleep apnea can be started before to the surgery.

If you are already using CPAP, please take your nasal interface (mask or cannula) when you go to the hospital. The hospitals can give you the CPAP, but your own mask will be more comfortable for you. You will sleep better that way.

Sleep Apnea can cause Seizures during sleep!

"If I am not on CPAP, my bladder releases! May be, I am having a seizure at that time" a pleasant 73-year-old lady with short, curvy whitish hair shared her insight with me, and she was correct.

The repeated cessations of respirations lead to frequent arousals and drops in the oxygen level. This reduces seizure threshold and precipitates seizure in susceptible individuals. Some of these patients may report bed wetting or tongue biting, but often just the tiredness and excessive sleepiness during the daytime. Quite often, they do not have daytime seizure episodes, just the sleep-related seizures, hence the possibility of seizures is not considered.

Our local neurologists have a high degree of suspicion and

refer patients, suspected of having nocturnal seizures, for an in-lab sleep study. Also, the patients on medications for a seizure disorder, who do not have daytime seizures, may benefit from a sleep study to make sure that they do not have sleep-related seizures. Talk to your doctor about it.

CPAP Improves Depression Symptoms Remarkably

My patients over the years have shared with me, "Doc, I am feeling great on CPAP. I am back to gardening, fishing, biking, camping, traveling. I now enjoy my work. My relationship has improved remarkably. We are back to sleeping together. Life is great!"

A study of 228 patients by Case Edwards and colleagues published in the Journal of Clinical Sleep Medicine does indeed confirm that the depression scores improve markedly with just three months of CPAP use. A total of 426 participants (243 males) were recruited for the study. Of 293 patients offered CPAP, 228 were compliant (mean nightly use > 5 h) over three months of therapy.

In those patients on CPAP, the depression scores went from 11.3 to 3.7, and the percentage of patients with severe depression score went from 74.6% to 3.9%.

The magnitude of change in the depression was similar in men and women. Antidepressant use was constant throughout.

The major findings of the study were that;

(a) depressive symptoms are common among patients referred for investigation of OSA;

(b) depressive symptoms are directly correlated with the severity of OSA;

(c) symptoms of depression, including suicidal ideation, are relieved by effective treatment of OSA with CPAP therapy; and

(d) These beneficial effects of CPAP are seen to a similar degree in men and women and are independent of the use of antidepressants.

The researchers concluded that the depressive symptoms are common in OSA and are related to its severity. They improve markedly with CPAP, implying a relationship to untreated OSA.

Hence, if you or your loved ones are feeling down and depressed, please talk to us at 574-534-9911 or your doctor and get tested for sleep apnea.

CPAP Helps Control Blood Sugar

"Why are my blood sugars high in the morning? I don't eat much at bedtime either," my patients have often complained.

Well, when you stop breathing repeatedly at night, your stress hormones go through the roof, and that causes your blood sugars to be high.

The study, published in the American Thoracic Society's American Journal of Respiratory and Critical Care Medicine, tracked 50 patients with both OSA and uncontrolled Type 2 diabetes. Some were asked to use CPAP masks, while the others were not.

After six months, the researchers found that the CPAP users had lower levels of insulin resistance and hemoglobin (HbA1c) levels — key markers of diabetes — than nonusers. Also, the CPAP group had fewer inflammatory proteins and other biomarkers associated with Type 2 diabetes blood sugar control.

Diabetic Kidney Disease May Get Worse with Untreated Sleep Apnea

Poorly controlled diabetes seen in patients with untreated sleep apnea leads to long-term complications.

Now, a metanalysis published in the February 2016 issue if Journal Sleep indicates that diabetic kidney disease (DKD) may get worse with untreated sleep apnea.

The researchers looked at two longitudinal, ten cross-sectional studies and seven studies for meta-analysis. Studies demonstrated significant associations between OSA and DKD in type 2 diabetes mellitus. A meta-analysis confirmed these associations.

This article gives you one more reason to get diagnosed and treated for sleep apnea. If you already are on CPAP, wear it every night, even when traveling.

OSA and Arthritis

A retrospective review of 105,000 patients with obstructive sleep apnea showed that these patients suffer from a higher risk of Rheumatoid Arthritis, Sjogren's Syndrome, and Behçet disease. OSA management is associated with reduced risk of RA.

I Threw My Father's CPAP Away

A patient in his late forties vented out his frustration about his father, who had recently started using CPAP.

Surprised by this unusual outburst, I just looked on waiting for him to elaborate.

"I used to visit him every week. He used to doze off in the recliner when I would talk about my business or my son! He just wasn't interested. I hated that. But, now, ever since you put him on CPAP, he has so much energy he is driving me crazy. Now, he is telling me how to run my business, how to raise my son. He goes to his every single soccer match and drives the coach nuts with his expert advice! I wish he could go back to being a sleepy head."

Well, this is a rare side effect of CPAP! Continuous Positive Airway Pressure keeps the throat open and allows sleep apnea patients spend enough time in deeper stages of sleep making them wake up alert and energetic. This renewed vitality can be an irritating problem for some.

Dr. Patel SR and his colleagues reviewed twelve trials of CPAP (706 patients with OSA) and published the findings in Archives of Internal Medicine. The meta-analysis found that CPAP reduced the Epworth Sleepiness Scale (ESS) score an average of 2.94 points more than placebo.

The ESS is a self-administered questionnaire designed by Dr. Murray Johns of Epworth Hospital in Melbourne, Australia. It provides a measure of a person's general level of daytime sleepiness or their average sleep propensity under various situations. It has become the world standard method for making this assessment.

Continuous positive airway pressure therapy significantly improves both subjective and objective measures of sleepiness in patients with OSA across a diverse range of populations. Patients with more severe apnea and sleepiness seem to benefit the most.

Patients have in fact over the years shared with me this improvement after they started using the CPAP.

"Doc, I did not know how sleepy I was until I started wearing CPAP."

"As if a hazy screen has been lifted off my eyes."

"I thought it was all stress and aging, but now I feel young again."

"I am thinking clearer. I am planning better. I am getting more done at work and home."

"I have so much energy that I don't know what to do with it."

"He is used to come home and doze off watching TV. Now, he does laundry, cleans the house, takes the garbage out..."

"I should have done this a long time ago."

In summary, if your family member is inattentive, unreceptive, lethargic and sleepy, please convince that person to get treated for sleep apnea. And after that be prepared to tactfully channel the resurgent energy!

Yes, CPAP Does Make You a Better Leader

Untreated OSA is associated with neurocognitive sequelae in memory, attention, and executive function.

Michelle Olaithe, BA (Hons) and Romola S. Bucks, Ph. D. (School of Psychology, the University of Western Australia, Perth, Australia) published, in the Journal Sleep, their meta-analysis of 35 studies looking at the executive function in OSA before and after treatment with CPAP.

The result indicated that the executive function is impaired in OSA compared to control participants.

People with OSA have difficulty shifting between tasks or mental sets, updating and monitoring working memory representations, inhibiting dominant or prepotent responses, they struggle with generating new information without external input or efficiently accessing long-term memory, and they have significant problems with Fluid reasoning or problem-solving.

All five domains of executive function showed medium to very large impairments in OSA independent of age and disease severity. Furthermore, all subdomains of executive function demonstrated small to medium improvements with CPAP treatment.

In summary, CPAP treatment of OSA can make you a much better leader. Indeed, my patients have over the years shared with me:

"I am thinking more clearly. My big picture skills have improved."

"I am more innovative, collaborative, and enthusiastic than ever before. I should have done this long time ago."

"I can fight off distractions and can stay focused on the task at hand."

"I was on the verge of getting fired. Three months later, I am being promoted!"

"I did not feel different when I started using CPAP, but when I missed it last week one night, I felt bad. I woke up achy and just not feeling right," an overweight truck drivers with severe apnea (apnea-hypopnea index of seventy-seven per hour) shared with me.

Can 6 hours' Sleep be Better than 10 hours' Sleep?

A middle-aged lady, an administrative assistant, told me that she would wake up exhausted even after sleeping for ten hours, but with CPAP, "I am ready to go after just six hours of sleep. This never happened in so many years! I used to wake up four-five times a night without CPAP, and now I sleep solidly for six hours and wake up full of energy."

When you spend more time in the deeper stages (N3 and REM) of sleep, you get more rest from six hours of sound sleep than from ten hours of poor sleep. This is the reason you should wear CPAP every night. Additionally, you should also avoid caffeine after 1 PM, alcohol within three hours of bedtime, and should exercise for half an hour a day.

Watch her brief video clip at
https://youtu.be/-8bGw0To168.

New Research Links Insomnia to Sleep Apnea

We do not associate insomnia with obstructive sleep apnea, but a recent study by Dr. Barry Krakow (Mayo Clinic Proceedings) showed the role of OSA in causing and perpetuating insomnia.

Krakow investigated 1,210 insomnia patients who were unable to fall asleep or stay asleep using sleep aids. Subsequently, 942 patients underwent overnight sleep studies, and 91 percent of those who completed a sleep study suffered from previously undiagnosed obstructive sleep apnea, a critical factor aggravating their insomnia.

If you suffer from insomnia, please talk to us or your doctor about a simple home sleep test to diagnose and treat obstructive sleep apnea.

I Lost My Job Because of You!

A tall, well-built truck driver in his sixties yelled at me with his finger pointed straight at me. I was stunned. He from time to time used to accompany his wife, who I had seen for decades for her asthma. I had always found him to be a mild mannered, soft spoken, pleasant man of few words. I understand that losing a job, more so in your sixties, can bring the worst out of you. I had tried best to help him comply with the state requirement, but he was stubborn, "I sleep fine. I don't have any problem. This is all a sham." He did not use his CPAP despite our best effort and lost his commercial license and his job.

In Indiana and in more and more states now, commercial drivers have to get screened and treated for sleep apnea.

Most drivers hate this. We understand their predicament, and we have designed a unique program to help them. We offer them a home sleep test with an identification tag. This test is accepted by the department of motor vehicles as it ensures that the patient did the test on the self and not on the dog! This test saves time and money ($300 versus $3000) compared to an in-lab sleep test.

We see these patients within days of the referral as opposed to several weeks if they were to call other clinics. Our medical assistants and billing specialists work with them patiently so that they can get back to work quickly but they have to do their part and use the CPAP regularly.

The average use of all nights should be greater than four hours and the percentage nights you used it for more than four hours is greater than 70%. If you do not meet this requirement, you may lose your job. So, commit yourself to the treatment. Work with our staff and your spouse. Try different interfaces. Do CPAP desensitization of anxious. Buy power accessories if you sleep in the truck. Good things in life are never easy. Do whatever you need to do, but please use CPAP. This way you shall keep your job, and will live longer and healthier. You may not like to admit but your CPAP may end up saving an innocent life on the road too.

Sleep Apnea Increases complications for pregnant women

New research from the University of South Florida has found that pregnant women with obstructive sleep apnea are five times more likely to die in the hospital during and shortly after pregnancy, compared with women without the disorder. The study also found that pregnant women with apnea also were more likely to suffer the severe complications of pregnancy, including severe high blood pressure, an enlarged heart and pulmonary blood clots.

Why does sleep apnea occur with greater frequency during pregnancy?

Hormonal changes of pregnancy relax your upper airway muscles causing a narrowing of the airway during inhalation, which in turn causes snoring and sleep apnea (repeated cessation of respirations lasting for ten or more seconds and robbing you of your deep sleep, causing severe daytime sleepiness and fatigue). Untreated, sleep apnea also increases the risk of gestational hypertension, preeclampsia, and low birth weight.

Untreated Sleep Apnea is Bad for Fetus Too

In the SLEEP journal, Blyton and colleagues report a series of three small studies of fetal activity in women with and without preeclampsia. They found objective evidence of reduced fetal movements in women with preeclampsia, many of whom had sleep apnea, and improvement in fetal movements following intervention with continuous positive airway pressure (CPAP). The CPAP treatment of these pregnant women may improve fetal well-being.

There has been a marked rise in publications in recent years showing that the obstructive sleep apnea is independently associated with gestational hypertension and preeclampsia. Unfortunately, a large proportion of pregnant women with gestational hypertension and preeclampsia appear to have unrecognized sleep apnea. Fortunately, our local obstetricians routinely screen their patients for sleep apnea and refer them to us promptly.

Sleep apnea linked to cancer death risk

Sleep apnea is associated with an increased risk for cancer mortality, study findings show.

"Remarkably, the association was stronger in relative terms than that of sleep apnea with mortality from all causes as well as that previously observed for cardiovascular mortality," told F Javier Nieto, from the University of Wisconsin.

Data on 1522 participants of the Wisconsin Sleep Cohort were studied. Of these, 222 had mild sleep apnea (apnea-hypopnea index [AHI]=5 to 14.9 apnea and hypopnea events per hour of sleep), 84 had moderate apnea (AHI=15 to 29.9), and 59 had severe apnea (AHI=30 or above or had a continuous positive airway pressure device present during sleep assessment).

Over a 22-year period, there was a total of 112 deaths, of which 50 were attributed to cancer, the most frequent being lung cancer (n=8).
After adjusting for age, gender, body mass index, and smoking, sleep apnea showed a dose-response relationship with cancer mortality.

Patients with mild apnea were 1.1 times more likely to die from cancer than individuals without apnea, while those with moderate and severe apnea were a respective 2.0 and 4.8 times more likely. This relationship persisted when patients treated with CPAP were excluded from analyses.
The researchers note that the risk of cancer mortality also increased in line with hypoxemia index severity. Participants in the top hypoxemia index category (11.2% of the night at less than 90% oxygen saturation) had a more than eight

times higher risk for cancer mortality than those in the lower category (0.8% of the night at less than 90% oxygen saturation).

This finding supports previous animal studies showing an association between intermittent hypoxia and accelerated cancer progression, and therefore hints at a mediatory effect of hypoxia on increased tumor tissue angiogenesis and resulting cell proliferation and tumor growth, the researchers explain.

They conclude that the diagnosis and treatment of sleep apnea in cancer patients may be indicated to prolong survival in cancer patients.

ADHD? Get Tested for Sleep Apnea.

A thirty-year-old obese night-shift worker was maxed out on his medicine for ADHD (Attention Deficit Hyperactivity Medicine). His family doc thought about sleep apnea as a potential cause for his excessive sleepiness and attention deficit. He ordered a home sleep test that showed apnea-hypopnea index of 104 per hour. CPAP auto brought it down to a normal of two per hour. His attention and memory improved. His hyperactivity disappeared. His doctor was able to discontinue Ritalin and lower the dosage of Vyvanse.

Sleep apnea has been shown to cause attention deficit and memory impairment in children and adults. The treatment with CPAP improves these.

For the First Time, We are Sleeping Together!

A pleasant forty-year-old lady was beaming with joy. "I may look like Darth Vader, but we are sleeping together now!"

She was troubled because her snoring had kept her spouse out of the bedroom for years. When she started sleeping with CPAP, the soft hum of CPAP replaced her stentorian snoring, and her husband started sleeping with her!

The health benefits of CPAP are so many that it is easy to forget about the benefit of sleeping together. Humans are social animals. They need company. They need touch, company, comfort, and warmth.

His Snoring Broke My Nose!

This is a true story that Dr. Chris Peers, an ENT doc, shared me with when I started my practice in Goshen in 1994.

A frail young lady consulted Dr. Peers for a broken nose. "I fell from my bed," she explained. On further questioning, Dr. Peers learned how this had happened. She was sleeping with her morbidly obese husband on their waterbed.

Her husband's stentorian snoring never bothered her as she was a sound sleeper. For some reason, the night of the incidence, his snoring was louder than usual. His snoring with each breath would keep on getting louder and louder as his upper airway became narrower and narrower. And then the throat shut off as it does in patients with sleep apnea. His struggle to breathe became intense creating giant waves in their waterbed. The airway finally gave up, and with a loud snort, he started breathing, but the Tsunami caused by this whole ordeal lifted this poor little lady off the bed into the air and finally on the floor face down!

Sleep apnea can be dangerous even for the spouse!

Are You Awake? I Don't Think So!

Several years ago, I was seeing a sleep apnea patient, a stocky man in his 50s, for a sleep study follow-up, "This is the sleep study we had ordered when we saw you last week…"

Before I could start explaining the sleep study findings, he interrupted me, "Doc, this is the first time I have come to your clinic. I wasn't here last week."

I was confused. Maybe it was a case of a mistaken identity. Perhaps, my staff had made a mistake. I stormed out of the exam room. I spoke to my receptionist and my medical assistant. It turns out that he, in fact, had been to our clinic the prior week (he had filled out all the necessary paperwork, and we had a progress note to prove his visit to the clinic) and was sent to the sleep center for a sleep study! But, he was so sleep-deprived that he was living in such a truncated level of wakefulness that he did not remember coming to our clinic at all.

For people like this, a quote shared by another patient comes true, "It feels like when I went to bed I was 18, and when I woke up I was 81!"

If you take care of your sleep, only then you can reach the

highest wakefulness, a state full of lasting energy, enthusiasm, vigor, and vitality. At that highest level of wakefulness, you can squeeze out one magical moment after another from this greatest gift called life. If not, then your whole life will feel like a fleeting moment.

Here, are the tips to help you improve alertness. You will learn more about these tips in the Section IV.

1. Get diagnosed and treated for sleep apnea.
2. Make sure your bedroom is dark, cool, and quiet.
3. Reserve your bedroom for sleep and sex only. Keep work-related items out of the bedroom.
4. Always maintain a consistent time to rise, even when circumstances prevent you from going to bed at your normal time. And, yes, that includes weekends.
5. Avoid consuming alcohol three hours before bedtime.
6. Avoid eating a heavy meal before bedtime because the process of digestion will interfere with falling asleep and may reduce the amount of deep sleep.
7. Sweat for sound sleep.
8. Stay away from caffeine, certainly after one o'clock.
9. Do not nap after two o'clock, and do not nap for longer than twenty minutes.
10. Develop a relaxing bedtime routine. Listen to the music. Read a nice book. Take a warm shower because the cooling off promotes sleep.
11. Pray on the pillow.

If you follow these tips consistently and religiously, only then you can be at the highest level of wakefulness and only then you can proclaim, "I am awake."

Transform Your Life and the World

Repeated cessation of respiration robs you of your REM (the dreaming stage of sleep). CPAP brings it back. You reach deep stages of sleep quicker every night and stay in the deep stages of sleep longer. Because of this, quite often the patients report dreaming when they start using CPAP.

If you learn to use these dreams to boost your creativity, you can change the world as your dreams contain a ton of revolutionary ideas.

Otto Loewi, who received the Nobel Prize in 1938 for his work on the chemical transmission of nerve impulses, wrote:

The night before Easter Sunday of that year I awoke, turned on the light, and jotted down a few notes on a tiny slip of paper. Then I fell asleep again. It occurred to me at 6 AM that during the night I had written down something most important, but I was unable to decipher the scrawl. The next night, at 3 o'clock, the idea returned. It was the design of an experiment to determine whether or not the hypothesis of chemical transmission that I had uttered 17 years ago was correct. I got up immediately, went to the laboratory, performed a single experiment on a frog's heart according to the nocturnal design, and completed my experiment.

Chemical structure of the benzene ring was also discovered during dreaming when the scientist saw a snake holding its tail in the mouth.

There have been at least two Nobel prizes, inventions of numerous medications, and a plethora of very successful stories, novels, and pictures attributed to the unrestrained creativity of REM (Rapid Eye Movement) sleep.

REM sleep, the most active state of our existence, has a hyperactive brain in a paralyzed body. Chaotic and incessant neuronal firings characterize REM sleep, leading to tremendous physiological activity and vivid dreams. Devoid of any constraints of time, place, or person, these vivid dreams spark innovation through out-of-the-world thinking. In the process, they help you create the world on your terms. With a bit of practice, you can tap into this innovative power of your REM sleep.

Wakefulness gives you access to 10 billion neurons, dreams to 90 billion.

Remember your dreams & then open your eyes.

By using electrodes thinner than our hair, MIT researcher Dr. Matthew Wilson recorded neuronal firing in a rat's brain as the rat ran a maze. He continued this recording when the rat was asleep. To his surprise, he found the neuronal firing during REM sleep was identical to that when the rat was awake and running the maze. Interestingly, these neuronal bursts during REM were even more intense than they were during wakefulness.

What's more, while dreaming, we do not respect anatomical barriers. (In fact, the rat would run through the wall.) So, during REM sleep, you are not just thinking outside the box, but also running outside the box without the risk of banging into the wall.

Dr. Sara Mednik, a researcher at the University of California, San Diego, administered a remote association test in which she gave participants three words and asked them to come up with a word that would link those three words; for example, given sixteen, heart, and candy, the answer would be sweet. After a nap containing REM sleep, participants produced a whopping 40 percent increase in correct answers, which strongly suggests that REM sleep enhanced the formation of associative networks and integration of unassociated information. This was after just a short nap containing REM sleep. Can you imagine the creativity after a full night of sleep containing a total of two hours of REM? Hence, if your teenager presents you with a tough problem, you should say, "Let me REM on it!" I am sure you would wake up with a creative answer that would surprise you and please your teenager. Maybe not, but sleep on a tough problem anyway!

"I think that these dreams involve a search for new and creative ways to put memories and ideas together," said Dr. Robert Stickgold of Harvard Medical School. "They can make associations that we wouldn't make when we're awake."

Here are a few helpful tips to help you use REM's Crazy Creativity to Transform Your Life:

Accept the fact that we dream every night. We may not remember our dreams, but with practice, we can learn to remember and even modify them.

In the afternoon and the evening, with positive emotions and unrestrained creativity, intensely contemplate on a major problem.

Ask for divine help by praying before retiring to bed. The Bible, in Matthew 18:23–26, says, "Have faith in God. I assure you: If anyone says to this mountain, 'Be lifted up and thrown into the sea,' and does not doubt in his heart, but believes that what he says will happen, it will be done for him." Praying helps us replace negative emotions, which are commonly associated with dreaming, with faith and optimism.

Keep paper and pencil on your nightstand. When you wake up at night to use the restroom, jot down what you were dreaming about and then go back to bed without thinking further. In the morning, look at your dream notes and elaborate on them.

Before opening your eyes in the morning, make it a point to ask yourself, "What was I dreaming about?"

If you use these tips, you will start tapping into the immense creative power of our brain. Also, remember this key point, even if you do not remember your dreams: They do occur every night, and they consolidate your memory and rearrange your information database, helping you think more clearly and, in the process, find a more creative solution.

I fly to Mars, enjoy a glass of Malbec while debating Abe Lincoln, hold the World Cup with Sachin, all in one dream. Why wake up?

Hopefully, I have convinced you to consider CPAP treatment. I do tell my patients that they should consider all the options before deciding about the treatment. In the next section, you will learn about the oral appliance, the hypoglossal nerve stimulation (pacemaker for the muscles of the throat), and various CPAP machines and nasal interfaces. This section also teaches you how you can get used to CPAP and how to derive the most benefit from your CPAP.

Section III

How You Should Use CPAP

A few of my patients would ask when I suggest CPAP for the treatment of their newly diagnosed sleep apnea, "What are my options?" Well, according to the guidelines published by American Academy of Sleep Medicine, the CPAP therapy is the most effective and preferred treatment of sleep apnea. If patients absolutely refuse CPAP treatment, then either the oral appliance (unless you have a severe sleep apnea) or the hypoglossal nerve stimulation are the options.

Should I Try an Oral Appliance?

"I have seen a commercial on TV about a mouth piece that can treat sleep apnea. This way I don't have to wear CPAP," my patients often ask.
Oral appliances have been approved as a second line therapy for patients with mild to moderate obstructive sleep apnea. They are customized by dentists, who are specially trained to treat sleep apnea.

While we have over 2000 patients using CPAP through our clinic as of August 2016, only 20 patients are on oral appliance. The following are the reasons:
1. Most insurances do not cover the cost of the oral appliance, which can range from 1000 to 12,000 dollars based on which dentist you go to.
2. My patients have complained about TMJ pain, gum irritation, and drooling at night. A few have also complained about the bite change as these devices pull the lower jaw forward to make the airway larger and tighter.
3. The oral appliances do not yet provide a way to monitor the effectiveness of the therapy.

These are the reasons, we recommend CPAP as the

initial therapy in all patients. After you have tried continuous positive airway pressure (CPAP) for at least 6 months and failed, only then you should try an oral appliance as the former corrects apnea (the cessation of respiration) and oxygen drops better.

Hours	2.9%
	28 days 6 hrs. 39 mins. 59 secs.
	7.9 cmH2O
ure	9.6 cmH2O
% of Time	9.5 cmH2O
Day	1 mins. 37 secs.

Home Test showed apnea hypopnea index

21/hr → 19/hr

oral appliance

"It was also causing me a few dental issues"

1.5

1/4/2017   EncoreAnywhere - version: 2.33.0.47   Page 1 of 3

nly one of several elements to consider when evaluating therapy effectiveness and is not a substitute for diagnostic data.

This patient, a soft-spoken retiree who volunteers at the local hospital, had tried an oral appliance for his moderate obstructive sleep apnea. As you can see that the oral appliance did improve his apnea a little, but the CPAP alone eliminated the apnea completely.

For snoring without the sleep apnea, an oral appliance will be the first choice, though.

Do remember that sleeping with an oral appliance, as discussed earlier, may aggravate your TMJ pain, cause drooling and gum irritation, and change your bite. You should also do a simple home sleep test with the oral appliance in place to make sure that the appliance is working.

What are the latest guidelines?

Well, the American Academy of Sleep Medicine (AASM) and American Academy of Dental Sleep Medicine (AADSM) commissioned a seven-member task force in the first half of 2015 to do a systematic review of the literature and develop recommendations.

What did they recommend?

1. We recommend that sleep physicians prescribe oral appliances, rather than no therapy, for adult patients who request treatment of primary snoring (without obstructive sleep apnea).

2. When oral appliance therapy is prescribed by a sleep physician for an adult patient with obstructive sleep apnea, we suggest that a qualified dentist use a custom, titratable appliance over non-custom oral devices.

3. We recommend that sleep physicians consider prescribing an oral appliance, rather than no treatment, for adult patients with obstructive sleep apnea who are intolerant of CPAP therapy or prefer alternate therapy.

4. We suggest that sleep physicians conduct follow-up sleep testing to improve or confirm treatment efficacy, rather than conduct follow-up without sleep testing, for patients fitted with oral appliances.

5. We suggest that sleep physicians and qualified dentists instruct adult patients treated with oral appliances for obstructive sleep apnea to return for periodic office visits— as opposed to no follow-up—with a qualified dentist and a sleep physician.

The oral appliance does have a place in the treatment of snoring and sleep apnea especially for the patients, who absolutely cannot tolerate CPAP. Please contact several providers in your area to get the lowest price and the best follow-up care.

Sleep on Your Side for Mild Apnea

If you have mild sleep apnea (apnea hypopnea index of 5 - 10/hr.) without excessive sleepiness, high blood pressure, depression, insomnia, or coronary artery disease or stroke history, then avoiding supine posture can help. This positional therapy is effective in patients, who have predominantly supine snoring and apnea.

You can achieve this by taking an extra size night shirt, a pair of socks, and two tennis balls. Put the tennis ball in each sock, trim out the extra length of the sock, and then sew this to the back of the night shirt such that these balls end up on your spine right between the shoulder blades. During sleep, when you roll on your back, the discomfort of these balls will roll you back on your sides. Elevating the head and the trunk to 30-60 degree can also help.

I will encourage you to get a repeat home sleep test with this night shirt to make sure that your sleep apnea is gone. You should also quit smoking as it irritates nasal and throat lining and makes sleep apnea worse. Weight loss will also help.

What About a Pacemaker for Sleep Apnea?

The US Food and Drug Administration (FDA) has approved a fully implantable neurostimulator to treat moderate to severe obstructive sleep apnea (OSA), but only as a second-line therapy.

The device, called Inspire Upper Airway Stimulation therapy, is manufactured by Inspire Medical Systems.

The implant helps keep a patient's airway open by stimulating the hypoglossal nerve during sleep in tandem with a patient's inspiration. The stimulation contracts upper airway muscles to pull the base of the tongue forward.

The FDA has approved Inspire Upper Airway Stimulation therapy specifically for patients with moderate to severe OSA who cannot use continuous positive airway pressure.

Inspire Therapy Overview

Inspire therapy is a small, fully implanted system that senses breathing patterns and delivers mild stimulation to maintain multilevel airway patency during sleep. Upper airway stimulation technology provides a first of its kind alternative for those suffering from obstructive sleep apnea who are unable to use or get consistent benefit from CPAP.

Inspire therapy is indicated for patients with the following characteristics: 22 years of age or older, have moderate to severe Obstructive Sleep Apnea (OSA) (AHI range from 20-65 with <25% central apneas), unable to use or get consistent benefit from CPAP, and free of complete concentric collapse at the palate. Inspire therapy has not been tested in people with BMI greater than 32.

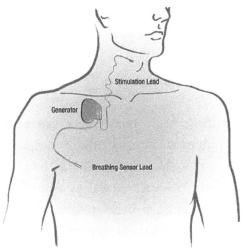

Stimulation Lead
Delivers mild stimulation to maintain
multilevel airway patency during sleep

Generator
Monitors breathing patterns

Breathing Sensor Lead
Senses breathing patterns

The Inspire system, as seen in the picture, consists of three implanted components including a small generator, breathing sensor lead, and stimulation lead, all controlled with the small handheld Inspire sleep remote.

Thoughtful patient selection, selective stimulation of targeted airway muscles, and optimal stimulation timing all play an important role in maintaining airway patency and improving patient outcomes.

For most patients, the Inspire system can be implanted during an outpatient procedure. Patients may experience some pain and swelling at incision sites but should be able to return to nonstrenuous activities after a few days. Approximately one month after implantation, patients return to their doctor's office where personalized stimulation settings are established and patients are trained to use the handheld sleep remote.

Adverse events reported in a clinical trial of the device included tongue weakness, dry mouth, pain, and numbness. The device is incompatible with having a magnetic resonance imaging scan.

This is an option available to you if you have severe sleep apnea and absolutely cannot get used to CPAP.

My Insurance Company Sucks

"Doc, should I room this patient right now? He has a follow-up appointment in a week to go over these results," Jennie, our medical assistant asked me as she handed me the home sleep test results.

This stocky young man, a UPS driver, had severe prolonged drops in his blood oxygen levels because of his severe sleep apnea.

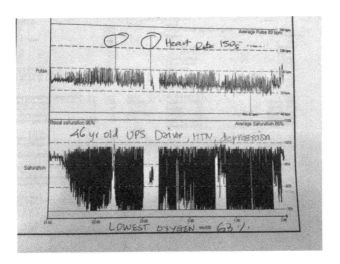

I saw him promptly and told Jennie to set him up on the CPAP ASAP.

"Well, we called his insurance when you were with the patient, and the insurance requires that we fax all the records to them and they will notify us of their decision in a week!" Dawn, another medical assistant informed me. These insurance companies usually have a nurse reviewing the records to delay or deny the services in most cases.

This is not the only time patients have to put up with the insurance companies. Sometimes, the sleep testing is not approved. At times, the deductible is too high. Often, the CPAP is not covered. Other times, the supplies are only partially covered. It goes on and on.

You will have to work with your employer, your physician, and your family to overcome these obstacles. Do whatever you need to but do get treated for sleep apnea. It will change your life. Your family members and your coworkers will thank you for it.

Should I See a Sleep Physician?

I recently noticed an old acquaintance at the receptionist's desk at my Mishawaka clinic. "Hey, how are you, my friend?" I asked.

"I am having difficulty with my mask," he answered.

This pleasant immigrant from India had a home sleep study done by a national company that mails the sleep testing equipment to these patients at the order of their family doctor. Then a report gets mailed out to the family doc stating that this study is positive and please prescribe CPAP at auto-titration setting of 5-20 cm. He received the prescription for CPAP and then started using it. He never saw his sleep test report. No one set down with him to explain him the findings, the need for the treatment, and the treatment options.

It turns out that this heavy set pleasant man had only mild apnea, which did not need such high pressures. Even more importantly, his apnea was so mild (apnea hypopnea index of only 6/hour) that just a few pounds of weight loss could have cured him of his sleep apnea. This is the reason every CPAP user see a sleep physician. The study below shows an additional reason for such consultation.

A study published in Journal of Clinical Sleep Medicine looked at various cues that the CPAP users found important from treatment initiation and adherence standpoint.

In this study by The University of Queensland, Australia, 63 adult patients diagnosed with OSA who had never tried CPAP were asked at 1 month as to why they started and persisted with CPAP use.

My sleep physician said that I should

My sleep physician was worried about my OSA

I was worried about the health consequences of my sleep problem

I was so tired all of the time

I was worried about my heart

My partner encouraged me to start using CPAP

My partner couldn't sleep because of my snoring

I was worried that I would have a car accident

These findings suggest that patients rate advice from health professionals (specifically their sleep physician) as very vital to their decision to commence on CPAP.

More than 80% of patients indicated that sleep physician-prompting to use CPAP and a perception of sleep-physician concern regarding patient's OSA were crucial cues to commence on CPAP.

The study suggests that a clear communication by the health professional is vital to patients in supporting treatment uptake.

I have seen quite a few patients (like the one mentioned above) who had a home sleep test equipment mailed to them by national company at the request of their family physician. Following the test, these patients will receive a call from a home medical company that their test is positive and their doctor has prescribed a CPAP for them to use. That is it. No one goes over the findings of the sleep test, the dangers of untreated sleep apnea, the difficulties they may encounter with CPAP initiation, and the possible solution to those difficulties.

In summary, consulting a sleep physician regarding your sleep apnea treatment will help your CPAP initiation and adherence. Hence, pick up the phone, make an appointment and talk to your sleep physician.

Should Buy an Auto CPAP or CPAP?

I was reading an in-lab CPAP study at Saint John's Hospital's sleep laboratory in Mishawaka. During the CPAP study, the technician titrates the pressure up to find out the final pressure needed to keep the throat open at all-times. That patient needed 14 cm as the final pressure. I told, Tom, the administrative director and a registered respiratory therapist, that I will put patient on an auto CPAP at 7 - 14 cm.

"What is with you and auto CPAP?" he inquired promptly.

"Why do you want the patient to get 14 cm pressure all-night long, when he needs lower pressure most of the night? The final pressure of 14 cm is needed only when he is in REM in supine position," I explained. This is the reason I prefer an auto-titrating CPAP over a fixed pressure CPAP.

An auto-titrating CPAP machine has a software that titrates the pressure in microseconds, breath by breath instead of giving you a fixed pressure all the time. You need the highest pressure when you are in REM sleep and on your back. You need the lowest pressure when you are in lighter stages of sleep and on your side. As you can imagine, it is easier to tolerate an auto CPAP certainly if you are on pressures higher than 10 cm.

The higher pressures can be difficult to tolerate. It can cause the swallowing of air leading to gassy stomach and belching on waking up. It can worsen claustrophobia. It may even lead to central apnea - cessation of respiration for ten-seconds or longer without the struggle to breathe unlike obstructive sleep apnea.

The autoCPAP also comes in handy when your pressure requirement changes because of weight loss or nasal allergies or aging. The only advantage of the fixed pressure CPAP is that it is usually cheaper by 200 or so dollars.

Our Patients' Favorite CPAPs

Which CPAP Should I Buy? This is the first dilemma facing you when you consider the treatment. The ideal CPAP should be light, quiet, easy to use, effective, durable, and elegant. It should have an adjustable humidifier to avoid nasal dryness and irritation. We also recommend an auto-adjusting CPAP (as opposed to a fixed pressure CPAP) as it can adjust the pressure breath-by-breath as opposed to giving you a constant pressure all-night long.

The CPAP should also give us the following information: How many hours did you use the CPAP for each night? Did you have residual apnea or hypopnea? Was there an air leak? What was the pressure required to keep your throat open?

Here, are the machines our patients have used and loved.

1. Dreamstation - Elegant Enough for Your Living Room!

We have used CPAPs made by Respironics for last twenty-five years and they have served our patients well. These are well-made, durable, state of the art machines that our patients have tolerated well. Their latest machine, Dreamstation has been especially favored by our patients because of its sleek looks, quiet operation, large display, and portability.

Other notable features include:
- A front-facing, easy to navigate display that can be seen sitting up or lying flat in bed
- An easy-to-clean, one-piece humidifier
- The EZ-Start helps you acclimate to the treatment, while SmartRamp allows you to fall asleep at a lower pressure
- A user-friendly troubleshooting feature that you can use and our staff can access remotely
- Integrated Bluetooth is standard on every Dreamstation
- DreamMapper feature provides goal-setting, helpful videos, and ongoing feedback to improve compliance

- Wake up to the summary of the night's use followed by a summary of the last 30 days of use

"So beautiful, I put it in the living room during daytime to show it off!" our first patient joked.

"I love the bright screen. The controls are simple too," another one commented.

"The unit is lightweight. The water tank is small."

"In the morning, I can look at the pressure needed to keep my respirations going."

"Love it. So quiet, I thought it might be OFF! Also love the ability to view the apnea hypopnea index and compliance."

We have approximately one thousand patients on this machine and they all love it. You can read more about other patients' comments on cpap.com. Our web site snoozeclinic.com too has patients' comments, but they are not as numerous as cpap.com as majority of our patients get CPAPs from our clinic in Goshen or Mishawaka and not from our web site.

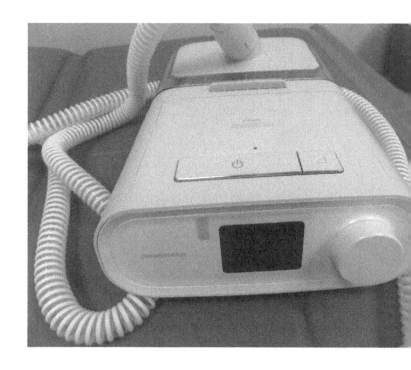

Here, are the few more features of this elegant device.

- We set all our Dreamstations with cellular modems so that we can monitor your usage and apnea hypopnea index to ensure success. Our medical assistants can also adjust the CPAP pressure remotely. You do not need to bring your CPAP for that.

- Dreamstations's EZ-Start automatic, personalized adjustments to CPAP pressure can help you gradually acclimate to the pressure.

- This machine's large display encourages compliance by giving you feedback every morning. It displays a simple trend of hours of use, apnea hypopnea index followed by a summary of last thirty days.

You can watch educational videos about this CPAP on our eStore at http://www.snoozeclinic.com

The Dreamstation sells for $ 868 on our eStore. A few websites hook you up by showing a lower price up front, and then during check out, add the humidifier and accessories to beef up the total. Our price, the lowest allowed by Respironics, includes a heated humidifier, heated tubing, and enrollment in our Free Filters for Life, a program we started several years ago when we saw numerous patients with allergies and sinus infections precipitated by clogged, old filters.

There are cheaper alternatives, but you should choose a durable machine from a reputable company when shopping for a primary machine. For our patients with financial constraint, one of the CPAPs mentioned in our travel section can be a consideration.

2. The ResMed AirSense 10 AutoSet for Her

This is a premium auto-adjusting pressure device for female patients. Of course, there is one for male patients with darker color and slightly different algorithm for auto-adjustment. It, just like the Dreamstation, includes an integrated humidifier, cellular connectivity and advanced event detection.

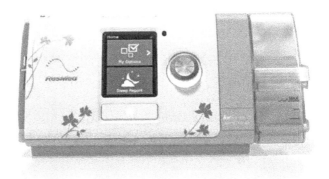

Other features of this sleek and smart machine include:

- Advanced event detection identifies central sleep apnea, respiratory effort related arousal and Cheyne-Stokes (waxing and waning breathing) events help us treat you better.
- AutoRamp™ with sleep onset detection delivers a low pressure to help patients fall asleep with ease. Once the patient is asleep, it comfortably ramps up the pressure to the prescribed level.
- The quiet Easy-Breathe motor makes for a peaceful environment for the patient and their bed partner. We have not had any complaint about the loudness so far.
- Expiratory pressure relief (EPR™) maintains the optimal treatment for the patient during inhalation and reduces pressure during exhalation.
- SmartStart™ allows the patient to start therapy by breathing in, instead of pressing the 'Start' button.
- AutoSet Response comfort setting offers gentler pressure increases and a smoother night's sleep to help patients with high pressure intolerance.
- Integrated humidification simplifies setting up the device and makes therapy easier.
- Using AirView™, we can access nightly therapy data, troubleshoot remotely (using the remote assist feature) and change device settings remotely.
- The user-friendly controls, intuitive interface and color LCD screen make it simple to navigate menus and customize comfort settings.
- Built-in ambient light sensor adjusts brightness of the screen based on the light in the room and turns off automatically. Patients love this auto-off feature.

So, research it and then buy the CPAP you can wear every

night.

3. Fisher Paykel's ICON+ Auto

This is the third on our list of our patients' favorites.

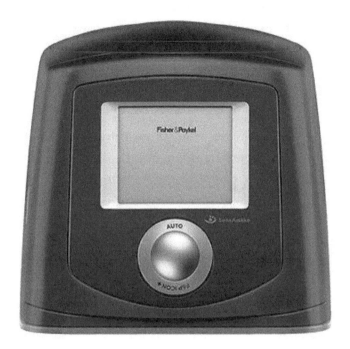

This boxy machine has a small foot-print on the nightstand and lacks any protruding parts or buttons. Our patients love its easy set-up, quiet operation, and diminutive size.

Other features include:
• SensAwake™ responsive pressure relief
• Built-In Heated Humidifier and ThermoSmart Heated Hose
• Auto-adjusting pressure for personalized treatment during sleep

- Info Technologies for flexible data communication options
- Contemporary and stylish design for bedroom appeal
- Forward-facing display with intuitive menu system
- Compact footprint including humidifier and power supply
- Combined smart technologies
- The versatile Auto CPAP device can be used as a titration and long-term solution for your patients. The flow-based auto-adjusting algorithm detects and effectively responds to flow limitation, hypopnea and apnea.

These are our patients' favorites. Research them online too and buy the one you like. If you live in Michiana, stop by and talk to our CPAP Geniuses for help.

Should I Choose a Mask or Cannula or Pillow?

You are recently diagnosed with Obstructive Sleep Apnea. Your doctor has prescribed a Continuous Positive Airway Pressure (CPAP) to keep your upper airway open and your respirations going.

You are overwhelmed though. You are anxious if you will be able to sleep soundly with CPAP. You are wondering if you should choose a nasal mask, or a full face-mask, or just a tiny nasal cannula to connect to your CPAP machine.

The choice depends on several factors.

If you are a mouth breather, a full-face mask may work better. The Amara View (released on June 15, 2016,) mask from Philips Respironics has become a popular choice of my patients as soon as it was available. It is lighter, smaller and has significantly fewer parts than leading traditional full-face masks. In fact, it requires just a single click to disassemble and reassemble the cushion and the mask frame for quick cleaning and replacement. Here is a 4-minute video clip where I explain the features of this mask.

https://youtu.be/rYE5cnJzY08

Smallest-Softest-Full Face Mask Amara View

The full-face mask works great for patients, who breathe both through their nose and their mouth. Amara View Full Face CPAP Mask is the smallest and lightest of all the leading full face masks, with the widest field of vision.

Here, are a few features of this popular full face mask:

- It is easy to use with one modular frame for all cushion sizes.
- The mask comes in Small, Medium and Large.
- Its innovative design prevents red marks, discomfort or irritation on the nose bridge.
- It is the smallest and lightest† of all leading full face masks.
- It offers the widest field of vision of all leading full face masks.
- It allows wearing glasses, reading, and watching TV.

The patient below used to use an older, larger full face mask, which gave him this skin lesion from the constant irritation. He was thrilled to put on Amara View!

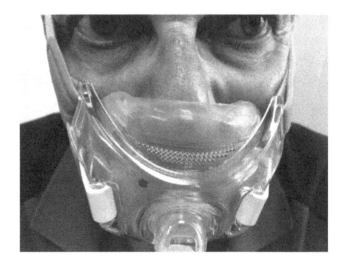

"I used Quattro FX for years with a band aid on my nose to prevent irritation. Doc showed me this when it came out in June. Have been using it for 2 months now. My skin irritation on the nose is gone. It does also feel less claustrophobic and restricting. The best full face mask so far!"

To watch my video about Amara View, please click on this link.
http://youtu.be/rYE5cnJzY08

If you breathe through your nose, a small mask that just covers your nose would work well. Fortunately, you have several options.

The Dreamwear
an interface so minimalistic even Steve Jobs would love!

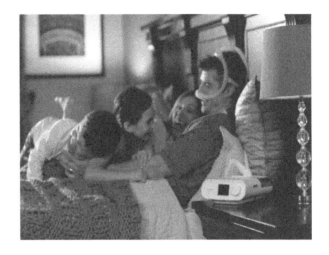

Our own Kim tried it for 3 nights and loved it. It is so simple, elegant, creative, and minimalistic.

"It does not go in the nose. It can't even irritate the bridge of the nose, " Connie, our CMA exclaimed.

"No more tubing hanging from the front of the nose," Deb noted as the tubing gets connected at the top of the head.

It is soft, light, minimal contact nasal mask that was quiet even at 20 cm of pressure.

The Dreamwear has quickly become the go to interface for our patients.

The older option is an Airfit N10 mask from ResMed. Our patients like this because of its cushion that fits comfortably on the face and the SoftEdge™ headgear, which minimizes facial marks.

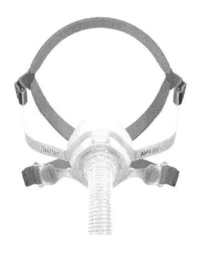

If you suffer from are claustrophobia, a nasal cannula may work better.

The picture below shows an AirFit P10 from Respironics.

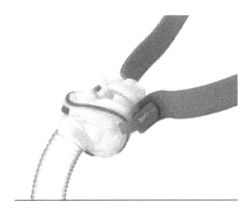

If your mouth opens up during sleep, you can always add a chin strap to your nasal mask or cannula.

Whether you choose a nasal mask, or a full-face mask or a cannula, remember to try several different sizes and shapes of that nasal interface. When you get a new interface, we suggest you put it on and keep it on without hooking it to the CPAP. Walk around the house with it on. Watch TV, or better yet, read a book. Let your face get used to the new interface and then go to the bedroom, hook it to the CPAP, and breathe slow and regular. Once comfortable, turn the CPAP on.

You may end up changing it over first several months until you find one that feels most comfortable. We do, at the clinic and on our eStore, offer a thirty-day exchange guarantee. If you do not like the interface after trying it for several weeks, just return it. We ship it back to the manufacturer and get a full credit. We do not reuse it.

The Elusive Search for a Perfect Nasal Mask

The nasal masks and cannula have improved remarkably since we started the sleep center in 1994, but they still have a long way to go before they can be near-perfect. Newer, softer, lighter, and smaller interfaces keep on coming out several times a year, still we are far from having one customized to your facial anatomy.

I do tell my patients though that we have do the best we can with what is available. It is far from being perfect, but much better than what it used to be. So, find something that you feel comfortable with, and stay with it. I will regularly update this book to introduce new machines and masks, hence keep on following my blog at SnoozeClinic.com. We will also be happy to send you the latest version of the eBook for free after you purchase the paperback or an eBook. Just send the request to me at Doc@SnoozeClinic.com.

My 5 tips for CPAP success

1. Nose is the key to success. Make sure that you don't have allergies and that your nasal passages are not inflamed.

2. Before you buy the mask, make sure it fits well and feels good on the face.

3. Be patient. It may take up to 6 months to get used to sleeping with CPAP.

4. If you have claustrophobia, try nasal pillows.

5. Use heated or cool mist humidifier to avoid dryness. Keep nasal saline spray (available over the counter) bedside and use it as needed.

You can also watch my video titled "How Not to Hate CPAP" on YouTube.

Patience Works

Over the years, I have had patients, who would swear that they can't see themselves sleeping with CPAP and the mask, but a year later, they will not sleep without it. It takes time to get used to wearing it just like when you start wearing a new pair of shoes or eyeglasses.

Look at the compliance report below of a reluctant patient. He did not use the CPAP much on the first night. He just wore the interface and watched TV or read the book without even hooking it to the CPAP machine. Next day, he used it for half an hour or so. He persisted and by the time he came to see me his compliance was perfect; his usage was six to seven hours every single night. He was feeling great too.

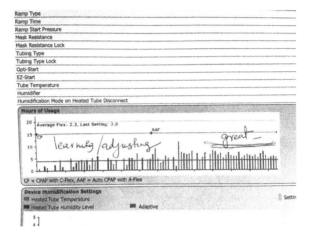

So, don't quit. Persevere. Give yourself time. Some relationships take time. Nurture it. Work at it. You will love it ultimately.

Seven Benefits of a PAP Nap Room

My wife and I visited the campus of Williams' Brothers in Washington, IN to learn how we can serve our patients better. Williams brothers run their family business in a compassionate, caring, and efficient manner. Julie, their CPAP specialist, a pleasant young lady in her 30s gave us a 2-hour long tour of their flawless operation.

"Let me walk you both to the parking lot," she said at the end of the trip. As we were walking through the large building, I noticed a room with a bed.

"We do all our CPAP set-ups in this room!" she proudly announced. Wow! So simple, and yet so helpful! We, like most providers, were setting CPAP up with patient sitting upright in the chair. How can one get an accurate idea of how the mask or the nasal cannula is going to feel when sleeping in bed?

Connie, our medical assistant, ordered a bed, mattress, bed covers, and other supplies from Amazon the very next Monday. Abbee assembled it right away in the examination room closest to the supplies room at our Goshen office, and the Nap Room was all set.

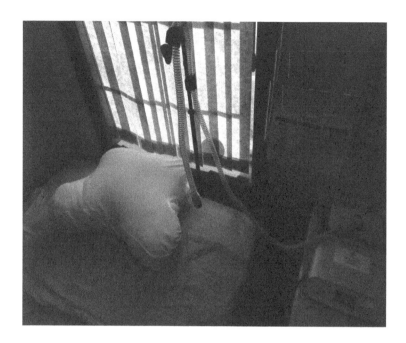

"Doc, we did our first CPAP set-up today," Connie called me excitedly when I was in our Mishawaka location. "He was euphoric. He told us he is just going to lay down, but won't sleep with the CPAP on. Well, we had to wake him up after half an hour, Doc!"

So, here, are the benefits of the Nap Room.

1. You can try the small mask or even smaller nasal cannula and lie down and see how it feels before taking it home.
2. You can also see if the PAPillow, the pillow with a cut-out to accommodate the mask or the cannula to minimize the air leak, feels right.
3. The interface may fit well sitting in the chair, but does it fit well when you toss and turn? You can learn that in the PAP Nap room.
4. The nap also allows you to check the Hose Suspension system to see if you need that or just want to use the headboard of the bed. This suspension system is very helpful especially if you toss and turn a lot. It prevents you from getting tangled up.
5. The PAP Nap also allows you to see how the humidifier and the control panel work.
6. The nap helps you gain the confidence that the CPAP, the tube, and the nasal interface work well. It reduces the anxiety associated with CPAP initiation.
7. The Nap Room also comes in handy during the follow-up visit if you are having difficulties with persistent snoring, apnea, or an air leak.

Well, we are excited about our Nap Room. Check it out when you visit us either in Goshen or in Mishawaka.

Why Should I Worry About Allergies?

When I inquire about their nasal allergy symptoms, patients often wonder and ask," I came here for sleep apnea treatment. What does that have to do with allergies?"

Studies (Respir Med 2000, Sleep 2003) have also suggested

that nasal congestion and symptoms are important reasons for abandoning PAP therapy or poor adherence to it.

The most scientific way to evaluate the allergy symptoms is to find out what you are allergic to by doing a simple and painless allergy skin testing using plastic bristles instead of needles. Once we determine the cause of your allergy symptoms then, we teach how you can minimize the exposure and thereby the symptoms.

You may have residual symptoms especially if you are allergic to dust, mold, pollens, or pet dander as these can be difficult to completely avoid. For these, taking allergy medications (Zyrtec or Claritin tablet, Fluticasone Nasal Spray, and Montelukast Tablet) can help.

For allergy symptoms refractory to the above treatment, immunotherapy, also called allergy shots (injecting dilute allergens into the skin on a weekly basis) can help.

If you alleviate allergy symptoms, then it will be easier to use CPAP all night long, every night. Discuss these with your doctor or call us for an appointment.

Depressed Despite CPAP? Treat Sleepiness

"I am not feeling better despite CPAP. I still feel tired and sleepy," a school teacher in her forties complained in a soft voice.

Untreated sleep apnea is associated with depression symptoms as we discussed earlier. The treatment with CPAP (Continuous Positive Airway Pressure) improves these symptoms in most, but not all patients.

In this multi-center prospective cohort study published in January 2014 CHEST journal, researchers evaluated 300 patients with OSA and depressive symptoms.

After an average of 529 days of CPAP therapy, the mean depression score decreased from 9.2 to 5.4, but 125 (41.7%) patients presented persistent depressive symptoms. The persistence of depressive symptoms was independently associated with persistent excessive daytime sleepiness, cardiovascular disease, and female gender.

Persistent depressive symptoms are strongly associated with Excessive Daytime Sleepiness. Active monitoring of depressive symptoms and of sleepiness is needed in CPAP-treated OSA patients. We routinely do Epworth Sleepiness Scale every visit. If the sleepiness scale is abnormal (greater than ten), we offer a stimulant medication called Nuvigil - armodafinil. This medicine, taken at the start of the day, helps boost alertness for ten to twelve hours. Unlike Ritalin, Adderall, or Dexedrine, this medicine does not raise blood pressure or heart rate. If you are feeling sleepy or depressed despite using CPAP, talk to us or your family physician about Nuvigil.

Don't Quit
Behavior Therapy Can Help

"Drugs do not work in patients who do not take them." Former Surgeon General C. Everett Koop had commented. Same is true for CPAP therapy. It will not improve your health and energy level unless you use it for seven hours every night even when traveling. It will take discipline, persistence, and team work between you, your spouse, employer, colleagues, and friends.

Some patients approach the CPAP therapy with strong negative thoughts and emotions. Some may suffer from claustrophobia, an anxiety disorder, or insomnia. The patients, who work nights, may also find it difficult to get used to CPAP. These are the patients, who benefit from behavior therapy.

The following behavioral interventions have been shown to improve CPAP adherence: frequent follow-up with the health care provider, intensive patient support and reinforcement, and cognitive behavioral therapy (CBT) plus education.

In a 2014 meta-analysis that included 13 small randomized trials examining supportive interventions to promote CPAP adherence, psychological support and encouragement were associated with increased CPAP usage (mean improvement, 50 minutes per night). In six randomized studies that included a total of 584 patients, CBT was associated with significantly improved CPAP adherence (mean improvement, 1.4 hours per night).

Frequent contact and follow-up with the health care provider who has expertise in treating sleep disorders is especially important during the first week of therapy to make sure that the CPAP settings are correct. General encouragement is offered and previously provided education (e.g., the importance of using CPAP each night) is reinforced. We routinely see patients at four weeks, and then three months after they start using CPAP. If they are doing well, then we see them every year after that.

Intensive patient support is best illustrated by a trial that randomly assigned 80 patients with OSA to receive intensive or usual support. Intensive support consisted of a three-night trial of CPAP in a sleep center, CPAP education at home (including the partner), and ongoing home visits once CPAP therapy had begun. Intensive support improved CPAP adherence (5.4 versus 3.9 hours per night), symptoms, mood, and cognitive performance at six months.

CBT is a structured psychotherapeutic method used to alter attitudes and behaviors. Look at CPAP not as a hindrance but as a life-sustaining and life-enriching intervention. I do remind them that it is a treatment though, just like the treatment for any other disease; diabetes, stroke, or even cancer. You may not like pricking your fingers, or daily exercise, or insulin injections, or chemotherapy for cancer, but you do it to treat the disease. The same is true for sleep apnea. I do have a number of patients, who dreaded the CPAP, but a year later, love it. "I can't go without it. It is a habit now."

PTSD and Sleep Apnea? Try These.

Treatment of Obstructive Sleep Apnea has been shown to improve anxiety, depression, and other symptoms of

Post-Traumatic Sleep Disorder but compliance with Continuous Positive Airway Pressure (CPAP) has been worse in these patients. My patients suffering from anxiety, depression, insomnia and similar symptoms do find it difficult to sleep with the CPAP.

If you or someone you know is suffering from PTSD and OSA, the following tips can help.

1. Get treated for PTSD. The treatment by your therapist or psychiatrist will improve your sleep quality and thereby your CPAP adherence, which in turn will help alleviate your PTSD symptoms. We request that you regroup and see them regularly.

2. Try a mild anxiety or sedative medicine. Talk to your physician about this. This will help you adjust to CPAP.

3. Practice Self-relaxation, meditation, and yoga. This can help reduce your anxiety about CPAP initiation. In our experience, these interventions are far more effective in the long run than the medications for anxiety or insomnia.

4. Use a small, non-intrusive nasal cannula instead of a large, bulky, suffocating mask. This will minimize claustrophobia and resultant anxiety panic feeling.

5. Attend a local CPAP support group. Studies have shown that such participation improves CPAP experience and adherence.

It can be difficult to get used to CPAP, but it is worth the pain. It not only improves your psychiatric symptoms, but would also improve your energy level and alertness. It will also reduce your risk of stroke, heart attack, high blood pressure, and drowsy driving death.

So, start using CPAP. Stay with it. Don't quit on it. Call us if we can help.

Team Up with a Buddy

Poor adherence to the CPAP therapy is common, with forty percent of patients being non-adherent to therapy when adherence is defined as greater than 4 hours of CPAP use per night.

A study of 39 patients by Dr. Parthasarathy and colleagues (Journal of Clinical Sleep Medicine – Volume 09-06) showed that partnering with an experienced CPAP user (peer buddy system) can improve the compliance significantly.

Participants in this study improved CPAP adherence by an hour or two each night when they teamed up with a buddy, who listened to them, understood their concerns, provided suggestions to solve their issues, and encouraged them to use CPAP every night.

A lot of our patients already have a coworker or two on CPAP, who provide periodic encouragement and support. If you do not have one, Find one at work, or church, or in your family. You can also ask your doctor or equipment provider about a support group that you can join. Keep on using CPAP, and then later on, be a buddy for a new user.

It Takes Two to Tango

Continuous positive airway pressure (CPAP) improves sleep and quality of life for both patients with obstructive sleep apnea (OSA) and their spouses, but adherence to CPAP therapy can be a challenge.

A study by Dr. Baron and colleagues at Northwestern University (the Journal of Clinical Sleep Medicine 2012) assessed the effect of spousal involvement in CPAP adherence in 23 married male OSA patients after the first week of treatment. At 3 months, 16 participants completed a second assessment of spousal involvement. Types of involvement assessed included positive (encouraging), negative (blaming), collaboration (working together), and one-sided (asking).

The result showed that collaborative spousal involvement was associated with higher CPAP adherence at 3 months.

CPAP adherence can eliminate excessive daytime sleepiness and reduce the risk of drowsy driving, uncontrolled blood pressure, blood sugar elevation, stroke, heart attack, congestive heart failure exacerbation, atrial fibrillation, and chronic lung disease exacerbation, but it can be difficult treatment to comply with the night after night.

You can help your spouse by saying:

1. I am happy you are trying to use CPAP.

2. I will set up the CPAP for you. Don't worry.

3. Hey, don't forget to put the CPAP on. You have been doing well this week.

4. It is for your health.

5. If you use CPAP every night, I will give you a gift!

Remember that this is a major lifestyle change and it can be difficult to adjust to CPAP. Your support can get him started on this life-saving treatment.

Anxious? Try Desensitization!

CPAP (Continuous Positive Airway Pressure) therapy for the treatment of Obstructive Sleep Apnea can be frightening for some. I have seen fear on their faces as soon as I walk in the exam room to discuss the treatment. For those patients, I have successfully used the desensitization technique described by Jack D. Edinger and Rodney A. Radtke in the Sleep Journal (Volume 16, issue 07).

This desensitization technique consists of the following five "steps":

1) Wear the CPAP nasal interface at home while awake for 1 hour each day without attaching it to the CPAP machine. You can watch TV, or read, or do chores with the mask on. It may look weird, but it does help you get used to CPAP. This is akin to trying a new pair of shoes in your house.

2) Attach the mask to the CPAP apparatus, switch the unit to the "on" position, and breathe through the mask for 1 hour while watching television, reading or performing some other sedentary activity.

3) Use CPAP during I-hour, scheduled naps at home.

4) Use CPAP during initial 3-4 hours of nocturnal sleep.

5) Use CPAP through an entire night's sleep.

When the patient reported performing one step for five consecutive days without anxiety, the patient was encouraged to move to the next, more difficult step. Therapeutic guidance was provided during five outpatient visits scheduled across a 3-month period.

I have noticed great success in several of my anxious patients with this technique. Patients feel empowered when making this life-changing transition. Their counterproductive anxiety turns into elation. Talk to your doctor about this and try it. You will sleep better and will wake up with more energy. Your health risks will also go down with the use of CPAP.

Will CPAP's Noise Keep My Spouse Awake?

"My spouse already has sleep difficulties; will my CPAP machine make her insomnia worse?" I reassure such patients that all the new models of CPAP devices are almost silent producing only 24 to 29 decibels.

Watch this video of a patient of mine sharing her experience. https://youtu.be/9i2mF-guUZ4.

"My husband loves the white noise of CPAP. He feels like it is the noise of the fan. When we were without the electricity, he could not sleep without that noise!" she told me.

How loud is 29 decibels? Here is a list of common noises and their decibel levels:

Normal conversation (60)
Refrigerator humming (40)
Whisper at 6 feet (29)
Whisper (20)
Calm breathing (10)

I further explain that most spouses find the soft, continuous, humming noise beneficial in helping them fall asleep, just like white noise would.

Some spouses have also shared with me that they sleep soundly knowing that CPAP is taking care of those dangerous episodes of cessation of respirations. They prefer this soft hum over stentorian snoring as the former represents continued breathing.

If you find a device's noise is bothersome, first check to make sure the CPAP's air filter is clean and unblocked.

If this doesn't help, have your CPAP supplier check the device to ensure it is working properly.

Also make sure that the CPAP mask is fitting properly as a large air leak from an ill-fitting mask can exacerbate the noise.

If the noise is still bothersome, try earplugs or a white noise sound machine to mask the noise.

Go through above checklist diligently and stay on CPAP.

I Pull Off My Mask in Sleep

"Doc, I put the CPAP mask on every night but wake up with the mask on the floor. I don't remember pulling it off," frustrated patients often share with me. I tell them that I never blame my patients for what they do once asleep, but there is no reason why they should not put the CPAP on in the first place. All I want you to do is put it on every time you get ready for sleep. You keep on doing this and one morning you shall wake up with it on!

In my experience, nasal obstruction is the commonest culprit. If your nose gets plugged during sleep, your mouth opens up, air leaks, your mouth gets dry, and you unknowingly pull the mask off. Studies have indeed shown that avoiding allergen exposure, and using nasal steroid spray at bedtime help keep the nasal passages open.

For such patients, we first do allergy skin testing followed by an intensive allergen avoidance education. We prescribe allergy medications like Zyrtec (Cetirizine) at bedtime along with fluticasone nasal spray to be used 2 sprays each nostril prior to putting the CPAP mask on.

If you still suffer from nasal obstruction, adding singular (montelukast) tablet as a maintenance medicine can help. Allergy shots (injecting measured dosage of allergens in your skin on a weekly basis) can alleviate your allergy symptoms and the need for allergy medicines. If you still cannot breathe through the nose, you may need an ENT consult.

A poorly fitting mask or cannula is another reason you may pull it off in sleep. Make sure you have the correct kind and size of the interface. You may have to try several different interfaces before you find the right one.

Other reasons for pulling the mask off in sleep include tight straps, skin irritation, excessive sweating, and too high a pressure. In autoCPAP mode, the pressure requirement is usually highest when you are in REM sleep and in supine position. You might be pulling off the mask when the pressure peaks. You can reduce this pressure requirement by losing weight or by getting younger! You can also try nasal steroid sprays at bedtime.

Talk to your doctor about these interventions and follow them. Be patient and persistent. Put on the CPAP mask every night and ultimately, one day, you shall wake with the mask on your face as opposed to your bed!

Air Leaks in my Eyes

Recently at our clinic, a sleep apnea patient in his 40s complained that he wakes up with red eyes because of the air leaking into his eyes.

The commonest cause of this is a poorly fitting nasal mask. If the mask is too big and reaches lower eyelid, it has the potential of leaking the air into the eye. This may not happen when you first put the mask on, but later on as the pressure on your CPAP machine increases, the air can leak out into the eyes.

A few patients have learned to readjust the mask at night, but can be an irritating problem if it occurs frequently. You can talk to our medical assistant and try a smaller mask or a different mask or even a nasal pillow to eliminate this air leak.

Dust, pet dander, and mold allergies can also irritate your

eyes. We can do a simple, painless skin testing and then can discuss strategies to minimize exposure to these allergens. There are over the counter allergy medications that can help. We also prescribe the allergy eye drops for our patients for nightly use.

Please do not let air leak or allergies prevent you from using CPAP. Talk to your doctor or to us and get them treated so that you can wake up with lasting energy and enthusiasm every morning.

Humidifier Helps Eliminate Dry Mouth

Humidification and early intensive education help improve CPAP compliance. Quite a few online stores promote CPAP machines without the humidifier to entice you with a lower upfront cost. We always encourage our patients to purchase CPAP with an in-built humidifier. You may not have dryness issue initially, but most likely will have it later on.

Even with humidification, a few of my patients complain that the CPAP is making their mouth dry, sometimes to a severe degree such that they cannot keep the CPAP on all-night long. These are the suggestions I have given to them over last 20 years of my practice.

1. Treat nasal congestion. Dry mouth occurs when you breathe through the mouth as your nose gets plugged up at night because of dust, mold, pets, or food allergies. Get checked out and treated for these allergies.

2. Check the side effects of your medications. Nasal decongestants, several types of blood pressure medicines, and antidepressants can cause dry mouth. Talk to your pharmacist and doctor to see if you can switch these medications or at least take them in the morning.

3. Use the humidifier attachment of CPAP. Dial up the setting on the humidifier of your CPAP machine. If you still suffer from dryness, you can also place an extra humidifier next to the bed.

4. Try nasal pillows. Patients sometimes can reduce this dryness by using nasal pillows instead of a full-face mask. You can add a chin strap if you are a mouth-breather.

5. Use nasal saline spray frequently. This is an over-the-counter product without any medicine in it, but is of great use as it not only moisturizes the nasal lining but also washes away the allergens and irritants. Keep the spray always on the nightstand. Use a couple of sprays in each nostril at bedtime and in the morning. You can use it when you wake up at night to use the restroom.

6. Consult an ENT specialist. This can help if you suffer from nasal obstruction because of a deviated septum or nasal polyps. Nasal obstruction will make you a mouth-breather, which in turn would make your mouth dry.

7. Stay hydrated. Drink water generously especially towards the evening to maintain good hydration.

If you follow these tips as applicable to your situation, dryness of mouth should abate. If it still continues to be a problem, talk to your doctor about other options.

Remember that an untreated sleep apnea increases your risk of uncontrolled blood pressure, elevated blood sugars, stroke, heart attack, and death. Please use CPAP every night.

I Have a Sore in My Nose

For immediate relief, you can try nasal saline gel. You can buy this over-the-counter from any pharmacy. Please dial up humidification setting on your machine. Switching to a heated tubing to moisturize the air can also help.

You can try a smaller nasal pillow. You can also switch to the Dreamwear interface as it does not go inside the nostril and hence does not irritate the nasal lining.

I Drool in My Mask!

A well-built man in his forties, shared with me this when I spoke to him about changing his mask to a nasal cannula.

Drooling can be irritating. It may disrupt sleep because of repeated awakenings. An open nose and a closed mouth can help minimize drooling. Nasal allergies and obstruction can increase the risk of drooling. I told him to try over-the-counter allergy medicines like loratadine tablet and nasacort AQ nasal spray at bedtime. I also told him to try a chin strap to keep his mouth closed during sleep. These interventions work in most patients. If you continue to have bothersome drooling despite trying these suggestions, talk to your dentist or consult an ENT physician for their recommendations.

I wake up bloated and gassy.

I do hear this complaint from time to time. The CPAP pushes air at a prescribed pressure to keep your throat open. In some patients, this air gets swallowed inadvertently during sleep and they wake up bloated and gassy.

These interventions can help.

1. The higher the pressure requirement, the higher are the chances of aerophagia (swallowing of air). If you are on a fixed CPAP of 20 cm, then you are more likely to swallow air compared to the CPAP of 10 cm. If you are on auto CPAP with variable pressure, then the chances of aerophagia goes down. You can reduce the pressure requirement even on auto CPAP by using nasal steroids (nasacort AQ or fluticasone 2 sprays each nostril at bedtime) and by weight loss. And as I joke with my patients, getting younger also lowers the pressure

requirement!

2. Caffeine relaxes the upper esophageal sphincter. Avoid caffeine.

3. Avoid a large meal at bed-time.

4. Put six inch blocks and raise the head end of your bed. This simple intervention is very effective in preventing acid reflux and gassy stomach.

5. Use Maalox or Mylanta at bedtime after checking with your pharmacist and doctor. This neutralizes the acid and gas in the stomach.

Try these. If you still feel unwell, talk to your doctor and see a gastroenterologist.

Sleep Apnea & Claustrophobia? Here is the Answer.

"My claustrophobia is so bad I can't ever wear make-up, Doc," a pleasant lady in her 50s shared her frustration with me before I can talk to her about sleep apnea and CPAP. Her BMI was 34. She had a narrow upper airway. Her blood pressure was up at 160/90. Her husband was sleeping in a separate room as her stentorian snoring kept him awake.

My patients with obstructive sleep apnea and severe claustrophobia are petrified at just the thought of wearing a bulky mask for use with their CPAP (Continuous Positive Airway Pressure) machine. Well, here is the answer to their prayers; a small, flexible, open, and wearable nasal interface, the Dreamwear from Respironics. Intensive behavior therapy as discussed earlier can also help.

My patients with claustrophobia have also found the following video extremely helpful in alleviating their anxiety about CPAP. The video is from a young lady with such severe claustrophobia that she could not even wear make-up. Now, she cannot sleep without her CPAP! Watch her at https://youtu.be/Ow0-Ock-aiQ.

CPAP & Night-Shift: A Tough Combination

Chronobiologist Franz Halberg coined the term "circadian," using the Latin circa (around) and diem or dies (day). Its literal meaning is "approximately one day." A person's circadian rhythm is an internal biological clock located in the hypothalamus portion of the brain. It regulates a number of biological, psychological, and behavioral processes over an approximate period of twenty-four hours.

Most of our bodily systems are subject to circadian variations. Bodily systems most affected by circadian variations include the sleep-wake cycle, the system that regulates temperature, and the endocrine system. The circadian rhythm is responsible for afternoon sleepiness and subsequent propensity for serious error and significant decline in our executive function. This afternoon dip in alertness is deeper and more prolonged in the presence of sleep debt.

This circadian rhythm also makes it difficult for the night-shift worker to sleep during daytime. This is especially difficult for the sleep apnea patients working nights. You have to make sure you follow good sleep habits religiously. You may need a sleep aid and an alerting medication.

If you have difficulty sleeping during daytime or difficulty staying awake during work despite these interventions, you may need to look for a day-shift work. Most of my patients do not like this as the day-shift work usually means a cut in the pay or problem with the child care (one spouse works days and the other works nights).

CPAP Use & Fibromyalgia

My empathy is with the Fibromyalgia patients. They feel exhausted and achy all-day; they can't sleep well at night anyway and now they have to use CPAP for their sleep apnea.

Even in the absence of sleep apnea, fibromyalgia causes non-restorative sleep characterized by frequent arousals and alpha intrusion (wakefulness like brain waves lasting for 3 sec or more). Their aches and pains too interfere with their sleep. Not only they have difficulty falling asleep and staying asleep, but also staying in stage 3 and stage REM sleep. The fragmented sleep makes their aches and pains worse.

The control of pain does improve deep sleep but it is difficult to achieve. To break this vicious cycle, it is absolutely essential that you follow sleep hygiene religiously.

Avoid caffeine completely. Avoid alcohol six hours of bedtime. Maintain a regular sleep wake schedule even on weekends. Exercise in moderation. Do water aerobics. Learn self-relaxation and mindfulness meditation.

See a Rheumatologist and discuss antidepressant medicine with sedating properties.

Follow with a sleep physician regularly to ensure CPAP compliance, sleep hygiene, and to exclude other sleep disorders especially restless legs syndrome as it can coexist with fibromyalgia.

Make Sure Your autoCPAP is Working!

We have seen Durable Medical Equipment companies drumming up their CPAP business by giving CPAPauto (These machines can adjust the pressure breath by breath to keep the throat open) to the patients after getting a home sleep test done by a third-party company that they have a working relationship with. Please remember that American Academy of Sleep Medicine (AASM) recommends that the patients with co-morbidities like diabetes, chronic lung disease, heart disease, and neurological conditions be referred for a CPAP study to find out the accurate pressure requirement instead of giving them a CPAP auto without such study.

The AASM also recommends that the patients, who are given CPAP auto, be seen by the physician in 4 weeks to make sure that the machine is taking care of the sleep apnea and that the patients is feeling better.

But, do these machines accurately and reliably treat sleep apnea? Dr. Zhu and colleagues tries to answer this question in the study published in the Journal of Clinical Sleep Medicine (July 2015). This study showed the auto-titrating continuous positive airway pressure (CPAP) devices are inconsistent in treating obstructive sleep apnea.

The study also raised a serious concern about the accuracy of the device compliance reports. These are the compliance reports that the sleep physician use to evaluate the treatment efficacy and to adjust the pressure on these machines.

Dr. Zhu and colleagues evaluated eleven commercially available CPAP devices on their reactions to obstructive apnea (cessation of respiration for 10 seconds or longer), hypopnea (abnormally shallow respirations), central apnea (cessation of respiration despite an open airway), and snoring.

Their results were startling.

In a single sequence of 30-minute repetitive obstructive apneas, only 5 devices normalized the airflow. Similarly, normalized breathing was recorded with 8 devices only for a 20-min obstructive hypopnea sequence.

Only five devices increased the pressure in response to snoring while only 4 devices maintained a constant minimum pressure when subjected to repeated central apneas with an open upper airway.

In the long general breathing scenario, the pressure responses and the treatment efficacy differed among devices: only 5 devices obtained a residual obstructive AHI < 5/h.

During the short general breathing scenario, only 2 devices reached the same treatment efficacy, and 3 devices underestimated the Apnea Hypopnea Index by > 10%. The long scenario led to more consistent device reports.

Device	Treatment Efficacy	Scoring Accuracy	Central Mechanism Detection	Snoring Detection	Patient Profile
D1	95%	67%	N	N	O
D2	81%	47%	N	Y	O, S
D3	100%	93%	N	N	O
D4	97%	N/A	N	N	O
D5	24%	99%	Y	Y	O, C, S
D6	94%	95%	N	N	O
D7*	84%	83%	Y	Y	O, C, S
D8	85%	91%	Y	Y	O, C, S
D9*	84%	94%	N	N	O
D10	96%	97%	N	N	O
D11*	57%	97%	Y	Y	O, C, S

Results were averaged over 2 tests (or 3 if * is indicated). Treatment of efficacy and scoring accuracy in the table were derived from the results of the long general scenario, in which snoring, "obstructive pressure peak" and cardiac oscillations were not simulated. Treatment efficacy, normalized as $TE = 1 - $ residual obstructive AHI / 38.6, in which 38.6 is the bench-simulated obstructive AHI in the long general scenario; Scoring accuracy, normalized as $= 1 - |\Delta$ Residual total AHI|, in which Δ Residual total AHI = (AHI report − AHI bench) / AHI bench × 100%; N/A, non applicable since the device data is not available for D4; N, negative; Y, positive. O, obstructive SDB profile; S, snoring; C, central SDB profile; D1, iCH Auto; D2, RESmart Auto; D3, iSleep20; D4, Floton Auto; D5, SleepCube Auto; D6, ICON+; D7, PR1 Remstar Auto; D8, S9 AutoSet; D9, DreamStar Auto; D10, Transcend Auto; D11, SOMNOBalance-e.

Ask your spouse if you snore with the CPAP on. The snoring or apnea may only occur in early morning hours when your REM sleep is longest and deepest. Unfortunately, this is the time your spouses' REM sleep will be deepest too. So, tell your spouse to look for snoring or apnea during that early morning trip to the restroom. Also, if you are feeling sleepy and tired despite using CPAP, you may need to do an in-lab CPAP study, or better yet do an in-office CPAP nap study, and then change the CPAP settings or the machine itself.

Sleepy Despite CPAP?

Majority of my patients feel more alert and energetic when they start using CPAP, but a substantial number of patients do continue to feel "no different from before." If you happen to fall in the latter group, follow these tips and talk to us or your doctor.

1. Ask your spouse if you snore or stop breathing with the CPAP on especially in the early morning hours. This would mean that the CPAP setting need to be adjusted.

2. Make sure you are using CPAP at least 7 hours every night. Studies by Antic et all published in Sleep journal (Volume 34, Issue 01) have shown that CPAP use of more than 7 hours provides the greatest chance of curing excessive daytime sleepiness.

3. Check with your pharmacist and your doctor to see any of the medications you take for your medical conditions can contribute to your fatigue, tiredness, or excessive daytime sleepiness. Further, ask them if these medications can be taken in the evening or at bedtime.

4. Make you sure you are not depressed. When I ask my patients if they are depressed, I often get, "I already am taking anti-depressant medication." I tell them it is still possible to have residual depression symptoms including fatigue, tiredness, and sleepiness.

5. If you continue to feel sleepy even after going through above checklist, talk to your doctor about Nuvigil, a stimulant medication.

I do stress to my patients that the CPAP use reduces the risks of stroke, heart attack, uncontrolled blood pressure, uncontrolled diabetes, and of drowsy driving death whether they feel better or not. CPAP in this regard is similar to cholesterol medication, which reduces the risk of stroke and heart attack, but does not make you feel better. You still keep on taking cholesterol pill to maintain your health. Same way, you should keep on using CPAP every night for seven or more hours.

Congestive Heart Failure? ASV Machine can be Harmful - a Study

On Wednesday, May 13, 2015, ResMed released a field safety notice for Congestive Heart Failure patients currently being treated for central sleep apnea syndrome with adaptive servo-ventilation (ASV) machine — a more sophisticated version of continuous positive pressure machine (CPAP).

In particular, if you have shortness of breath, chronic heart failure and a reduced left ventricular ejection fraction (LVEF ≤ 45% — a measure of your heart's squeezing function), using ASV may be harmful. Based upon the early results of the randomized controlled SERVE-HF study, for this particular at-risk population, there is a 33.5% increased risk of cardiovascular death, compared to control patients who are not on ASV therapy (absolute annual risk: 10% in ASV patients vs. 7.5% in control group).

What Should You Do?

Only you and your physician can determine the best course of action.

Work with your family physician, your cardiologist, and your sleep doctor to determine the best course of action. We first make sure that you do have Central Sleep Apnea. We have ordered for several patients a repeat diagnostic sleep study to determine this. Your cardiologist may repeat an echocardiogram to assess your ejection fraction — the squeezing function of your heart. If you do have central sleep apnea and a weak heart, Other evidence-based therapies for CSA might include CPAP or oxygen, but long-term outcome studies for these therapies are not conclusive either.

Please remember that these findings do not apply to Obstructive Sleep Apnea and to the use of Continuous Positive Airway Pressure use, which in fact have been shown to reduce the risk of uncontrolled blood pressure, stroke, heart attack, atrial fibrillation, drowsy driving, and sudden death.

PAPillow for air leak

A few patients, who like to sleep on their side, have complained about the mask sliding off a beat as the face rests on the pillow. This can cause a significant air leak leading to eye irritation, and more importantly, apnea because of the pressure leakage. The noise of the air leak can also wake up the patient and the spouse too.

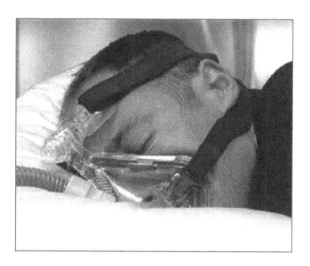

To solve this problem, we had Bob, one of our medical

assistant's husband, try a PAPillow and he loved it from the first night.

Like Bob, I too got an opportunity to try it, without the mask though as I do not have sleep apnea. It was on a beautiful August day, when I rode my new bike to work. Because of this, I could not drive home for a quick lunch, and a power nap. The staff room was noisy as the drug rep was still teaching the crew about a new sleep aid.

I decided to open a pillow and nap in one of the exam rooms.

The pillow was wrapped in a soft thin plastic that was easy to tear. The cover was neatly folded and felt smooth and soft. Putting the cover, I realized that it was cleverly made to fit the pillow perfectly without distorting the pillow or leaving any excess cloth on the sides.

I put the pillow on the exam room table and put my head on it. It did not feel too firm as some of my patients have commented. I rolled on my right side, and even though I did not have the CPAP mask on, I could imagine how that recess can help the CPAP users. The fabric felt soothing to my face. I fell asleep to the relax chant of Aum only to wake up like a new person twenty minutes later when my timer went off!

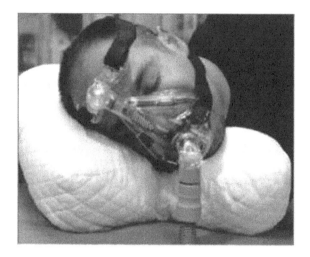

This pillow, as shown in the above picture, has a concave cut-out on each side to allow the face mask rest in the air as opposed to pushed aside by the pillow. A quite a few patients have tried this pillow and have loved it. The pillow supports your face without even touching the mask! A very simple, yet clever design!

This pillow prevents mask leaks and the soreness from the pressure points.

You can purchase it from our clinic or our eStore at http://SnoozeClinic.com.

That is my story. And here, is what the manufacturer has to say!

Proudly made in the USA, the unique patented design has resolved compliance issues for tens of thousands of CPAP users. PAPillow™ is the original CPAP bed pillow created by CPAP users, for CPAP users developed in 2000 and launched to the world in 2002.

PAPillow™ has a long history of proven performance because of the high standard we adhere to. Our patented design, top quality components including the quilted side panel, are what set PAPillow apart from all others.

You will find that PAPillow provides proper support for neck and head, accommodates both left or right side sleeping.

The hypoallergenic synthetic down fill provides support while maximizing comfort at the same time. The quilted side panel prevents the edge from collapsing. A hundred percent cotton interlock-knit fitted pillow case is included with your order.

The pillow is machine washable and cool dryer safe.

Here, are the routine care instructions:

For optimum life, fluff daily and refluff occasionally in a tumble dryer at warm setting for 10 minutes.

All commercial and home laundry detergents are approved for use as long as the manufacturer's instructions are followed. Always balance the load and use water temperatures not to exceed 120 F. We recommend enclosing the pillow in a mesh laundry bag and using a front loading large capacity washer on gentle setting. Do not wash a damaged pillow.

Tumble dry at temperatures not to exceed 120 F. Pillows may take a few hours to dry depending on your dryer. For additional agitation place clean tennis balls in with pillows. Keep drying until all synthetic feathers feel light and fluffy. If necessary, air dry (cool down) for an additional 30-60 minutes depending on your dryer. Caution! Never allow pillows to sit in a hot dryer after the drying cycle is over. Use the cool down cycle or remove pillows immediately from dryer.

Surface wipe with neutral detergent and lukewarm water. Do not use bleach. Surface rinse and dry thoroughly. Do not machine wash or dry.

Surfaces wipe with a quaternary solution at the recommended dilution ratios. You should first test the fabric with the solution you are using to be certain that the fabric is performing as required. Under no circumstances should a phenolic-based cleaning agent be used.

The PAPillow is bacteria and fungus resistant, stretchable, fluid proof, and stain resistant.

In short, if you are a side sleeper, then check this pillow out. It will help you sleep better.

Why Change Mask Cushions and Pillows?

"Don't fix it if ain't broken!" a patient reluctantly shared with me when I asked him about his CPAP supplies renewal.

The recommendations for the supplies renewal from the manufacturers and DME companies appeared to me to be motivated by personal gain. Now, I have become more and more religious about advocating and even insisting that all my patients change them as recommended.

To make my point, I will share the story of an Amish patient in his 50s. Using CPAP, he felt better, but not all the way. His pretreatment apnea hypopnea index was 43/Hour. On his CPAP compliance report, it was 13.5/Hour, which is abnormal. The recommendation is to keep it less than 5/Hour. We like to keep it close to 0/Hour!

Why was he having residual apnea? At least, in part it was the air leak from not changing his mask cushion! Take a look at the following compliance report in the right half of the image.

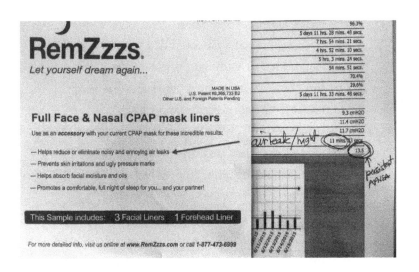

This patient got rid of his air leak just by changing the mask cushion.

He also added the RemZZZs mask liner as he was getting some skin irritation where the mask cushion was touching the skin. These mask liners have become a favorite supply our patients pick up from the clinic routinely. Below, are a few details from the manufacturer.

Simply incredible - Incredibly simple

As you may know, both CPAP and respiratory therapy haven't always been therapeutic for many people. Fortunately, that was before RemZzzs®. You can think of it like this: RemZzzs® will help you and your mask become friends. This is possible because our patented design acts as a barrier between the skin of your face and the silicone of your mask's cushion, virtually eliminating all of the most common problems associated with wearing a CPAP mask. And best of all, it's very comfortable! But comfort is just the tip of the iceberg. RemZzzs® can:

- Promote healing of suspected deep tissue injury.
- Greatly reduce or eliminate noisy and annoying air leaks.
- Prevent skin irritations and ugly pressure marks.
- Help absorb facial moisture and oils.
- Assist with comfortably holding your mask in place.
- Allow for the use of bedtime facial products.
- Promote a comfortable, full night of sleep… for you and your partner!

Along with all of the benefits above, RemZzzs® can save you a lot of time. Manufacturers' recommend cleaning your mask at least once a day, every single day. Talk about an extra day-job! With RemZzzs®, our naturally absorbent fibers act as a barrier between you and your mask, keeping oil and moisture away from the silicone cushion. The result is you spending less time cleaning your mask, and spending more time actually enjoying all of its benefits.

It is made of 100% breathable cotton knit. The RemZzzs® is shaped to fit the area of a patient's face which comes in direct contact with a respiratory and/or CPAP mask;

including bony bridge of nose, forehead, and cheeks.

Most of our patients routinely use these RemZzzs because of these reasons. Too bad, the insurances do not cover these must have accessories.

The CPAP Tube Choked Me!

"I do not thrash around in bed much, doc. This is the reason I was surprised and startled when the hose got tangled around my neck and choked me hard enough to cause a bout of coughing. It scared my wife too in the middle of the night."

John, a thin tall man in his early 60s, is a sleep apnea patient, who wore his CPAP every night, even when traveling. He was one my first patients when we started the medical practice several decades ago.

Until this point, I had not used the hose suspension system in my patients. This episode highlighted the importance of such a system to avoid such problem. We started offering the hose suspension system from Hose Buddy to our patients starting with John.

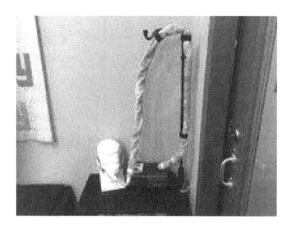

The picture above is from our waiting room in Mishawaka. The triangular base is placed between the box spring and the top mattress. The hose is secured with the velcros supplied with the system. The picture shows the optional hose cover, which our patients use to prevent condensation. They also like the looks of the hose cover. You can order the hose cover by clicking here.

The system is easy to set up. It is adjustable in height and width. John loves using it. It also prevents condensation from trickling down to the mask and the mouth.

Should I Buy a Travel CPAP?

A patient of mine, John Miller, a chubby and pleasant plant manager at a local rubber factory in Goshen, Indiana, while on a Caribbean cruise, woke up in the middle of the night with a racing heart rate and flutter in the chest. It went away quickly and only to wake him up an hour later, only this time with more severe and persistent symptoms. Worried, he woke his wife up, who got their son from the next cabin. They took him to the medical clinic in the lower deck of the ship. His heart rate was up at 160/min. He was in atrial fibrillation, a condition characterized by irregular and rapid heart rate. He had this condition so long ago that he had forgotten about it, until this episode. The cruise doctor came, started him on intravenous medicine, a blood thinner, and kept him in observation for 24 hours.

John had ignored his wife's advice of taking his CPAP on this trip. During his study, without CPAP, his respirations during sleep will cease for 15-20 seconds at a time with oxygen levels dropping into 70s (the minimum oxygen level required for the body to work without stress is 90 percent). The recurrence of atrial fibrillation is directly related to the severity and duration of such drop in oxygen level.

Because of this and other less dramatic events my patients have shared with me over last couple of decades, this is what I tell my them:

"If you want a healthy and uneventful vacation, you should take your CPAP with you."

"Don't you want to feel alert and energetic so that you can enjoy the beautiful sights and sounds while visiting exciting places?"

"Do you want to doze off when your grandkid is making a castle on the beach?"

Sometimes, I joke with them, "Your CPAP machine is like your cute pet. It loves to travel. Take it with you on your trips!" or "Do you want to keep everyone awake with your stentorian snoring?"

Some of them ask me if they will have a problem getting the CPAP through the security at the airport. "No, I haven't had any patient in 22 years of my practice, who had a problem." Quite a few security personnel are on CPAP themselves. I even have heard one of them saying, "Those with CPAP machines, please go to this line," at the airport in Denver. In our local airport in South Bend, Indiana, I have seen a sign directing the patients with CPAP to a separate lane.

If my patient is traveling to an international destination, just to be on the safe side, I do write a note stating, "Jane Miller is under my care for obstructive sleep apnea, for which she needs to carry and use CPAP machine every night during sleep. Please call me for questions."

John's CPAP was old, big, bulky, and loud. But, if you have one of the newer CPAPs, which are small, light, and quiet, you can choose to take that with you while traveling. You can take it without the added bulk of humidifier. If you suffer from a dry mouth without the humidifier, you can take a nasal saline spray with you and use it several times a night to moisturize your nose and the back of your mouth. You can also keep a glass of water with a straw on your lamp stand for night-time sips.

A lot of my patients though like the convenience of a travel CPAP so that they do not have remove their primary CPAP from their set up in the bedroom. On coming back from their trip tired, they do not have to unpack the CPAP and reassemble the set up in the bedroom. These travel machines are very light (less than a pound) and small such that they make a convenient travel companion. They stay on the lamp stand of a motel, hotel, or a small cabin of a cruise.

So, review the available travel CPAPs, choose one, buy one, and travel in style and in health.

Which Travel CPAP Should I Buy?

Here, are the top five travel CPAPs for under $500.

I will start with my patients' all-time favorite travel CPAP.

1. The Transcend Auto miniCPAP. The cost of this fabulous CPAP on our eStore is $425.

It is the smallest, light (weighs less than a pound), quiet (26.6 dB), and fun to use especially with auto-adjusting pressure. It is a cool looking little machine that will dazzle people at the airport security line or on the lamp stand when sharing a room!

Here, are the salient points from the manufacturer:

- Transcend AUTO is a fully featured APAP with EZEX pressure relief. The Auto continually monitors you're breathing to adapt to your changing therapy needs. Transcend EZEX technology provides pressure relief on exhalation for more breathing comfort.

- One of its biggest differentiators from any other CPAP on the market, Transcend has two battery options, a solar battery charger and a DC mobile power adaptor, giving unmatched power options that support therapy on the go.
- From your desktop, up to the cloud, TranSync™ makes it easy for CPAP users to track and share their therapy data.
- Transcend AUTO is a fully featured APAP with EZEX

pressure relief. The Auto continually monitors your breathing to adapt to your changing therapy needs. Transcend EZEX technology provides pressure relief on exhalation for more breathing comfort.

- Small, fully featured AutoPAP
- Transcend EZEX™ pressure relief technology
- TranSync compatible
- Most innovative & portable APAP in the world
- Weighs less than one pound
- QUIET

Transcend is extremely quiet for its small size. Engineered with a vibration-free blower, Transcend only makes 28 dB of sound.

One of its biggest differentiators from any other CPAP on the market, Transcend has two battery options, a solar battery charger and a DC mobile power adaptor, giving unmatched power options that support therapy on the go.

From your desktop, up to the cloud, TranSync™ makes it easy for CPAP users to track and share their therapy data.

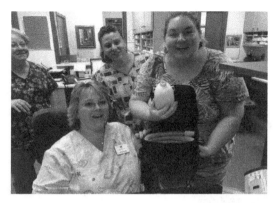

Our front
office staff is excited when we gave our first Transcend
CPAP out!

Don't forget to watch this fabulous video from Peter Rowe
about his use of this device in the Himalayas!

http://youtu.be/0opX3jjXAhw

2. The Apex XT Auto CPAP Machine

XT series is one of the smallest CPAP in the market. Its palm-sized and lightweight design lends itself well to travel. However, it delivers the same effective therapy as the larger machines, includes useful features like easy-to-adjust ramp settings, automatic altitude adjustment, leak compensation and data collection by SD card. And now, enhanced pressure stability and the clinically proven algorithm make the New XT series even more comfortable, with the introduction of the pressure relief function. The cost at our eStore is $385 at the time of the publication of this book.

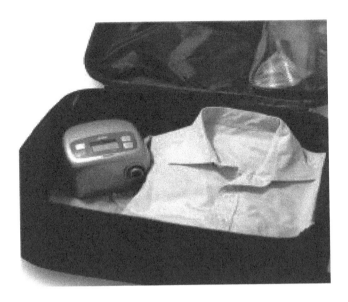

XT's palm-size design makes it easy to be packed into carry-on luggage.

It has a built in power supply, an easy-to-use interface, and an SD card for recording and sharing your usage data. You can also retrieve usage data using the USB port. My patients have also enjoyed the built in clock and alarm function, especially during traveling.

It is a quiet machine with a noise level of 28 dB, slightly louder than a whisper. This becomes important when sharing a room during your travel.

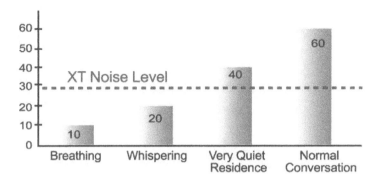

The APEX auto-CPAP device employs proprietary, precision algorithms to optimize treatment by adjusting air pressure to the lowest, most comfortable levels, while still maintaining effective, appropriate therapy. Clinical trials have consistently demonstrated how the APEX auto-CPAP can reduce RDI levels below 5.0 and increase SpO2 levels above 95%, while allowing patients to rest comfortably throughout the night.

We have observed this machine's flawless ability to cure our patients' sleep apnea during their follow up visits. I am yet to remember a patient on XT Auto with a significant residual apnea.

When traveling abroad, there is no need to use the converter for Apex's CPAP systems can accept 100-240V, 50-60Hz, without any special adjustment. An international plug adapter may be required to make the power cord compatible with the power outlets of that country.

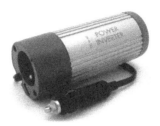

The XT series CPAP system doesn't have the DC capability so it can't be powered by a battery or a car adapter. However, it can be used with a DC to AC inverter to power on (only CPAP, not the Heated Humidifier)

The air filter should be cleaned at least once every two weeks or more often if this device is operated in a dusty environment and replaced with a new one every six months.

Question? Please drop us an email at Doc@SnoozeClinic.com and one of our medical assistants will get back to you within a working day.

Happy Travels

3. The XT Fit CPAP Machine

This is a budget-friendly ($199) version of the XT Auto CPAP from Apex manufacturing. It is ideal for patients, who are on a lower CPAP pressure or who do not mind the constant high pressure. Most of my patients whose pressure requirement is less than 15 cm are able to tolerate this fixed pressure CPAP.

The size is same as XT Auto machine. Even though it lacks the auto-adjusting feature, it does have the convenience of the ramp feature, leak compensation, and compliance reporting.

When traveling abroad with XT Auto, there is no need to use the converter. This CPAP can accept 100-240V, 50-60Hz, without any special adjustment. An international plug adapter may be required to make the power cord compatible with the power outlets of that country.

4. IntelliPAP AutoAdjust Travel CPAP Machine with SmartFlex

This machine gives one more option to choose from when shopping for a light, quiet, and comfortable travel CPAP. It is a little pricey at 490 dollars.

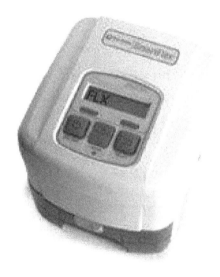

The IntelliPAP AutoAdjust unit can be operated in both conventional CPAP and AutoAdjust modes.

AutoAdjust features include:

- Automatic pressure adjustment based on event density and type
- Adjustable definition of apnea and hypopnea (percentage and duration)
- Adjustable upper and lower pressure limits
- Adjustable delay setting for up to four hours
- Automatic detection of mask conditions and ultra-sensitive snoring detection

This device offers patented SmartFlex® technology which offers three comfort settings, with each setting equating to an exact 1 cm H20 drop in pressure upon exhalation.

DeVilbiss SmartFlex also features patented Flow Rounding which changes the slope of the pressure waveform during the transition from prescription pressure to the SmartFlex setting and vice versa. This enables a smooth transition and decreases the likelihood of waking the CPAP user.

There are six levels of flow rounding with level 0 having the steepest slope and quickest transition and level five having the gentlest slope and slowest transition.

5. Z1 Travel CPAP Machine

This travel machine costs $700 for the auto version and $575 for the fixed pressure version. The manufacturer claims that it is the smallest, lightest, most integrated CPAP machine available.

The New Z1 Auto™

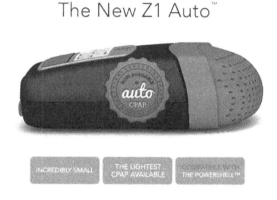

The Z1® is the lightest CPAP machine available anywhere. At only 10 ounces it is a great everyday machine that is also ideal for travel.

A few patients have complained about the noise, but the manufacturer reports that it only makes 26 dB of sound during operation. This noise is comparable to a whisper from a distance of six feet.

At an added cost, the Z1 CPAP system offers an optional integrated battery system called the PowerShell™ shown below. It delivers a full night of cord-free power on a fully-charged battery.

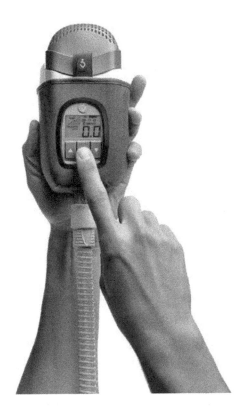

Slip the Z1 CPAP into the PowerShell™ and you have a full night of cord-free sleep. You can purchase extra battery modules to enjoy several nights of cordless use while camping or hiking. It can also operate as a failover power source.

These are the favorites of my patients. Use a CPAP even when napping and traveling.

I will regularly update this book to introduce new travel machines and masks, hence keep on following my blog at SnoozeClinic.com. We will also be happy to send you the latest version of the eBook for free after you purchase the paperback or an eBook. Just send the request to me at

Doc@SnoozeClinic.com.

If You Use CPAP Only for 6 Hours
You are at Increased Risk for Heart Attack

A study in this month's SLEEP journal shows that men who habitually sleep 6 hours or less have a reduced secretion of tissue Plasminogen Activator, body's natural clot buster, which dissolves the clot in coronary arteries. This puts short sleepers at an increased risk of heart attack and stroke.

Here are my 5 tips to help you fight this when you cannot get 7-8 hours of sleep every night because of work or family responsibilities.

1. When you cannot get a sufficient amount of sleep, it is absolutely vital that you get maximum percentage of deep sleep by using CPAP and by following sound sleep hygiene. A lot of the time we not only get insufficient sleep but also poor quality sleep.

2. Invest 15 min into a strategically placed (usually between 1-3 pm) power nap. It cannot only improve your productivity, but also reduce your heart rate and blood pressure, thereby reducing your risk of heart attack.

3. At work, try to walk more than you stand, and stand more than you sit. Conduct walking meetings instead of traditional sitting ones. If you sit at the desk a lot, invest in laptop stand and do the same work by standing.

4. Make salad for lunch a routine. Enjoy nuts and fruits as snacks in the afternoon.

5. Look at the problems with optimism and positivity. Studies have shown that people who interpret workplace events with optimism have a reduced risk of heart attack. Make sure you use CPAP for seven hours on an average.

Waking Up Repeatedly at Night?

I was seeing an executive in his 50s for a routine CPAP follow-up. He was using CPAP for 7 hours and 32 minutes every night. His sleep apnea was well-controlled with only one per hour of shallow respirations as seen in the following compliance report. But he was waking up repeatedly at night and feeling tired during the daytime. He was irritable, grumpy, and nervous all the time.

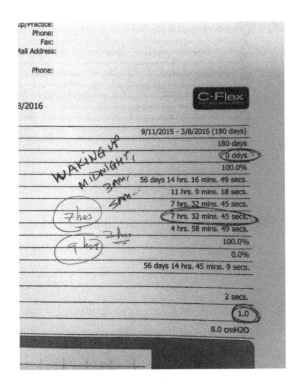

The reasons were obvious:

1. He was working only 40 hours per week, and yet was not exercising at all. We talked about a daily exercise of 20-30 minutes doing water aerobics or a stationary bike to minimize his knee pain. This should reduce his awakenings and should improve his deep sleep percentage.

2. He was worried about his parents who were recently placed in a nursing home. We talked about writing a journal every night in the living room outlining problems and solutions. Once he closes the journal, he will stop thinking about it.

3. He was getting frustrated at night when he could not fall back asleep. We talked about progressive muscle relaxation to use when he wakes up at night.

4. He was staying in bed for 9 hours from 9 pm and 6 am. Most Americans need 7 hours of sleep on an average. The reason for his sleep difficulty is obvious; if you need 7 hours of sleep and spend 9 hours in bed, your brain will be awake for 2 hours no matter what. Because of this reason we talked about sleep consolidation. He will go to bed at 10 pm and see how he slept.

5. He would switch to decaf coffee even in the morning. Caffeine has a duration of action of 24 hours. A cup of coffee in the morning may cause repeated awakenings at night in a sensitive individual.

6. He will not consume alcohol after 7 pm. Alcohol may put you to sleep, but it will rob you of your deep sleep and it will cause frequent awakenings.

You can try these interventions to minimize your awakenings

and get more REM sleep. This will improve your energy level and your executive function the next day.

Can't Fall Back Asleep? Do What Your Doc Does!

"Doc, sometimes I wake up in the middle of the night, and can't fall asleep so I take my CPAP off."

I see this on the compliance reports often that you are using CPAP for three or four hours and then taking the CPAP off.

Well, there are times even a sleep doc can't fall asleep! This happens most commonly prior to a big trip or sometimes after a page from the hospital or a phone call from the sleep lab. I used to get frustrated when I could not fall back to sleep. I would worry about the busy day next day, which in turn would make matters worse.

Same thing would happen the night before a long and challenging day at work, I sometimes find it difficult to relax at bedtime. As a result of this, I find it difficult to fall asleep, which makes it difficult for me to enjoy my work the next day. To counteract this, I have learned and successfully used progressive muscle relaxation.

The technique is simple:

1. Lie flat on your back in bed with your arms resting at your sides.

2. Slowly breathe in and out.

3. One by one, tighten and then completely and pleasantly relax each muscle, starting with the scalp muscles and moving down to the face muscles (eyes, lips, cheeks), neck, shoulder, chest, arms, abdomen, back, legs, and all the way to the toe muscles.

4. Repeat this process several times until you achieve complete relaxation.

The goal is to achieve a sense of complete weightlessness through total physical relaxation.

Ready to relax even more? Learn Shavasan (Shav means corpse, Asana means posture). You may initially find it morbid and dark, but it certainly takes the whole relaxation process a lot further. During Shavasana, you not only aim for a total physical relaxation, but also for a complete and total mental inertia.

How can you achieve Shavasan? Well, you go through above mentioned four steps, and then try to achieve a state of the compete thoughtlessness. You basically try to lay there like a dead person; no muscle tone, no mental activity, no awareness of external or internal activity! This is what makes this the toughest of all Yoga postures. But, with practice and patience, you will keep on improving. Keep trying and you shall sleep better.

Then I work on my racing mind. I practice complete detachment (Vairagya). I observe these thoughts as a third person. They arise and they subside. I do nothing with them. I give up all the worries, desires, expectations, and anger to Almighty, to the Higher Power, and I just lay there completely relaxed.

This is called Savasana, which literally means "corpse posture." When I do this, I get the physical, mental, and spiritual rejuvenation despite being awake.

I may fall asleep; I may not fall asleep. I do not worry. I do not care. Sleep is a natural phenomenon. If it comes, it comes. If it doesn't, it doesn't. I don't care. I trust the Lord. I have been through tougher times with little sleep in the past. I can do that again with the help the Lord.

Besides improving your deep sleep, the progressive muscle relaxation and Shavasan provides the following benefits:

a decrease in heart rate and the rate of respiration
a decrease in blood pressure
a decrease in metabolic rate and the consumption of oxygen
a reduction in general anxiety
a reduction in the number and frequency of panic attacks
an increase in energy levels and in general productivity
an improvement in concentration and in memory
a decrease in fatigue

Well, I hope you don't have difficulty falling asleep, but if you do, I urge you to try Savasana. If you find it beneficial, share this information and spread the wealth!

Section IV
Good Sleep Habits Lead to an Alert Life

I use CPAP every night, but still wake up tired

We hear this from our patients from time to time. They expect CPAP to make them feel alert and energetic despite their poor sleep habits; a sedentary life, caffeine consumption, working in bed, alcohol use close to bedtime, and a poor sleep environment to name a few.

We spend 1/3 of our life sleeping. This investment can pay handsome dividends provided we follow sleep hygiene. If you ignore sleep hygiene then you shall fail to capitalize on this investment and as a result, will wake up exhausted. You will run out of energy in the afternoon, and end up living a suboptimal life. It does not make sense to use CPAP and ignore other habits that can give you more of deeper (N3 and REM) sleep. This is comparable to a diabetic patient taking insulin regularly but eating sweets and leading a sedentary life.

Create a Sanctuary for Sleep

The first rule of sleep hygiene is to create a sanctuary for sleep. Get TV, laptop, Smartphone and iPad out of your bedroom. If you need to keep your phone in the room for any reason, keep it face down. Put dark drapes on the windows. Keep your bedroom dark, cool, and quiet. Make sure your mattress is comfortable. Keep the wall color dark. Try nature sounds to put you to sleep. Aromatherapy can help too. And hang a poster on the wall that will set the tone for sound sleep. Here are my favorites from http://www.allposters.com.

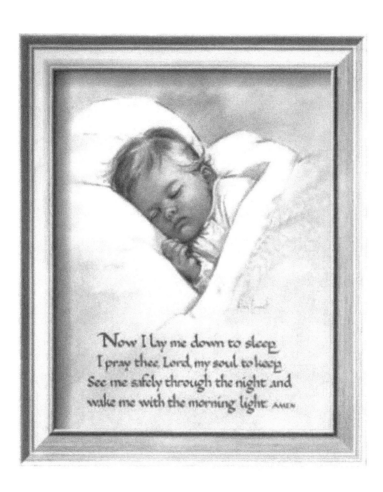

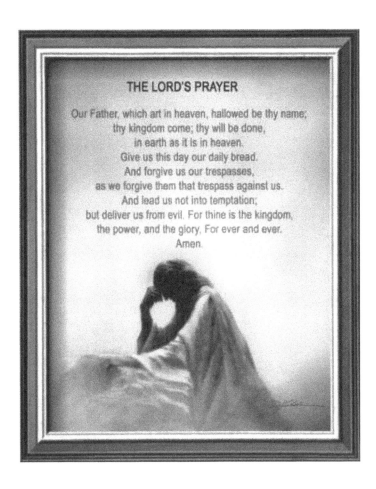

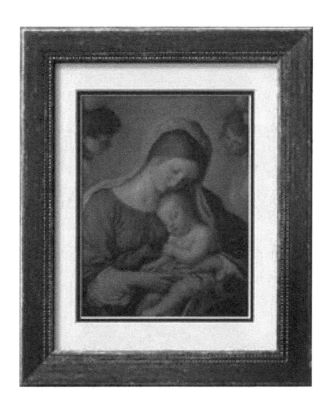

Sleep Like Bats!

Pineal gland, a tiny structure located at the base of the brain secretes melatonin, a sleep-promoting agent. Based on our internal rhythm, this secretion starts in the evening approximately two hours before sleep onset and peaks two hours before wakefulness. The melatonin release is extremely sensitive to bright light. Light emanating from even a tiny phone screen can reduce this secretion and prevent you from falling asleep and getting enough deep sleep. Here, are a few tips to help you maximize your internal melatonin secretion.

Here are a few tips to help you maximize your internal melatonin secretion.

1. Choose dark drapes or blinds for the bedroom windows. You can also apply a black film over glass windows to block out light completely. A dim nightlight to guide you safely to the restroom at night is acceptable as long as you are not facing it in your favorite sleeping position. Also, choose a night-light with the lowest brightness. Ideally, the bedroom should be so dark that you should not be able to see your outstretched hand!

2. Turn the alarm clock away and keep the brightness to a minimum.

3. Completely turn off all the electronic devices including stereo, satellite boxes, TV, laptop, iPad, and others. Again my preference, as we have discussed before, is not to have these devices in the bedroom at all. If you use them in the evening, please use them outside the bedroom and with lowest possible brightness to maximize melatonin secretion.

4. Sport those cool-looking designer sunglasses while driving

home in the evening or during outdoor activities in the backyard. Your pineal gland will love you for that.

If your spouse needs nightlight, please use one with the lowest brightness. I also suggest you try dark and comfortable eyeshades. These eyeshades come in handy when trying to sleep in those not-so-dark hotel rooms.

Pray After You Put the CPAP On!

Do you ever wake up tired and sluggish even after a good night's sleep? This can occur because of the negative emotions, which get amplified during REM (the dreaming stage) sleep. Most of us do not remember our dreams, but they occur every night and leave a mark on our mood. The studies have shown that anxiety, fear, and other negative emotions predominate during our dreams. Can we change this? Can we infuse our dreams with positive emotions? Can we use this to our advantage by praying on the pillow? Well, try it tonight and find out.

Here, are a few of my favorite bedtime pillow prayers.

If anyone says to this mountain, 'Be lifted up and thrown into the sea,' & does not doubt, it will be done.

Wake me up at the end of a fabulous dream.

As I sleep, Lord, fill up my vast subconscious with hope, happiness, joy, and bliss. And then wake me up with the highest level of consciousness.

As I dream tonight, my Lord, take me to the enchanted corners of every galaxy.

As I sleep, my Lord, replace hatred from my subconscious with faith and love.

Lord infuse energy & enthusiasm in every neuron of every brain tonight.

Praying before sleep eliminates negative emotions while praying after sleep prepares you for the day. It infuses energy, enthusiasm, and optimism. Praying with your afternoon nap recharges your spiritual engine, while on-the-go prayers maintain your equanimity during the challenges at work. Try this tonight on the pillow and then, tomorrow, off the pillow.

Love Coffee?

I was seeing a middle-aged patient, husband of my kids' elementary school teacher, for snoring, daytime fatigue, and tiredness. He already had a sleep study which was negative for sleep apnea but did show increased arousal index (number of times brain waves show wakefulness activity lasting for 5-10 secs). Arthritis, sedentary life, fibromyalgia, alcohol usage, and periodic leg movements of sleep can increase the arousal index. I explained him the sleep hygiene instructions, and reassured him that he did not have sleep apnea. As I was leaving the exam room asked him what he did for fun. "I grind coffee beans," he replied with a beaming smile on his face! He would enjoy a flavorful cup of strong black coffee every night!

"I don't have a problem falling asleep though," he insisted fearing my recommendation. After initial hesitation, he did slowly taper his caffeine down. His fatigue and tiredness disappeared soon after he eliminated bedtime coffee and switched to decaf coffee in the morning!

Here are a few more tips from your sleep doc:

1. Avoid coffee after 1 pm. "I am going to switch his coffee to decaf coffee without telling him," a nine-year-old cute girl with colorful braces and a baseball cap on her blonde hair told me when I was getting on her dad's case about drinking coffee all-day.

2. Smell, sip and enjoy decaf coffee same way you enjoy a glass of good wine. Drink mindfully.

3. If you are a morning person, you do not need coffee in the morning. Go with a glass of orange juice or a cup of decaf coffee.

4. If you are not a morning person, enjoy a nice cup of coffee in the morning to kick start your day. My personal favorite though is "bed to bike" routine. Jump on the stationary bike as soon as the alarm goes off. Do not let your mind talk you out of it. You can read on the bike, watch the news, or check emails (you can get a very nice laptop stand which can work with the bike or even with your treadmill. I bought one from http://www.airdesks.com, and I love it.)

5. The surest indication for a strong cup of coffee is drowsy driving. The coffee here can be lifesaving. Go ahead. Enjoy it. You have my full support. Power nap can also provide similar benefit though without robbing you of your deep sleep (REM sleep and stage 3 NREM sleep.)

6. Never drink just to drink. You will not take medication just to take medication. Caffeine is no different. Drink it for a reason; to maximize alertness while driving or attending an

important meeting.

7. After-dinner coffee is suicidal for sleep. I feel like getting up and yelling a loud NO when the waiter offers coffee to the guests after the dinner. Please help me stop that life-robbing tradition.

8. Avoid caffeine before and during menstruation as it worsens both the PMS (Premenstrual Syndrome) and also the insomnia associated with menstruation.

Learn to enjoy caffeine judiciously and selectively.

5 Reasons to Drink at 5!

It provoketh and it unprovoketh. - Shakespeare

Alcohol arouses sexual desire, but retards performance. It has a similar effect on sleep; it induces sleep, but it is a poor quality sleep marked by frequent arousals. It also makes snoring and sleep apnea worse by making the upper airway more collapsible.

My friends did not like it when I insisted that they should not drink within three hours of bedtime. Because of this, I changed my message: Start drinking early! They love it!

1. Alcohol within 3 hours of bedtime causes frequent awakenings and arousals, which will rob you of your deep sleep making you wake up tired, achy, and grumpy the next day.

2. Decreasing level of alcohol causes a state of hyper-arousal leading to an early morning awakening.

3. Alcohol relaxes upper airway muscles making your snoring and sleep apnea worse. If you are on a fixed pressure CPAP, this might be a problem as alcohol increases the pressure needed to keep your throat open.

4. Alcohol, being a diuretic, causes frequent nighttime urination thereby robing you of your deep sleep further by sleep disruption.

5. Alcohol relaxes upper esophageal sphincter (a tight band of muscles at the upper end of our food pipe) thereby making acid reflux worse which further interrupts our sleep.

Hence, enjoy a glass of Malbec at 5 PM and then sleep sound from 10 PM to 6 AM.

Using CPAP When Suffering from Insomnia

Insomnia refers to the inability to fall asleep or stat asleep or both. Depression, anxiety, and Psychophysiological (learned) insomnia are the commonest causes of insomnia.

"I am on depression medicine already, Doc," is the comment I usually hear when I mention the possibility of depression as a cause of insomnia. Well, it does not mean that your depression is gone. You can still have a partially treated or unsuccessfully treated depression causing insomnia. Please, talk to your family doc and get your depression treated well.

The psychophysiological insomnia refers to continued difficulty falling asleep, even after the initial stressor has long gone. The whole experience of going to bed reminds us of the difficulties we had during those stressful days. We dread going to bed. We are anxious and therefore more awake when we try to go to bed. We keep on worrying about the impact this will have on our life the next day.

Recognize it. Learn self-relaxation. Progressive muscle relaxation is an easy-to-learn and immensely useful technique. Reassure yourself that one or two bad nights are not going to paralyze your executive abilities.

Learn and follow these suggestions for sound sleep when suffering from insomnia:

Create a sanctuary for sleep. Bats sleep sixteen hours a day because they are in cool, dark caves. Make your bedroom dark and cool, too. Use darker colors on the wall.

As discussed earlier, hang relaxing pictures on the wall, ones of beautiful landscapes, gorgeous mountains, Buddha meditating, or the Baby Jesus sleeping in his mother's lap.

Have dark blinds or heavy, dark drapes that block out light completely. Make sure the mattress is comfortable. If you like a firm mattress and your spouse prefers a soft one, then a Sleep Number mattress is the answer.

Do the best you can to minimize noise. Soothing white noise can help promote deep sleep. Based on your preference, you can use the sounds of ocean, nature, or running water to achieve a similar effect. A recent study showed that keeping your head cool also promotes sleep.

Learn a relaxing bedtime routine. A warm shower can help, because cooling off after a shower can be conducive to sleep. Listening to soothing music can calm your anxious nerves. A glass of skim milk and cookies can also help, because milk contains tryptophan, a naturally occurring sleep-promoting agent.

Go to bed only when sleepy, not just tired.

Most patients need six and half to seven hours of sleep. If you spend nine hours in bed, you will be awake for two hours no matter what you do. Consolidate your time in bed. Do not spend too much time in bed.

Read a relaxing book. Listen to soothing and calming music. If you are not asleep after approximately twenty minutes or so, get out of bed. This will prevent formation of learned insomnia. Do something relaxing in the living room. Return to bed only when sleepy.

Keep the clock face turned away. Looking at a clock at night will stimulate your brain.

Don't fight Mother Nature. Even on weekends and even after a bad night, get up at the same time every morning. Use your inbuilt circadian rhythm to your advantage in this fight against insomnia.

Avoid taking naps while going through insomnia treatment. If you must take a nap for emergency purposes, restrict it to twenty minutes or less before two o'clock for as long as possible.

Use your bed only for sleep and sex. Ignore your laptop or smartphone completely when in the bed. When working on your laptop in the evening, keep the screen brightness to a minimum. Watching TV in bed will stimulate your brain, too. Get rid of the TV in the bedroom.

Recognize that exercise is the best ally of sound sleep. It

helps us fall asleep quickly, stay asleep longer, and get more REM sleep. Even after a rough night, get twenty to thirty minutes of exercise anytime during the day, as long as it is not just before retiring to bed.

Do not eat a big meal just before bedtime. The digestion process and acid reflux will both interfere with sleep.

Avoid caffeine. Caffeine has a twenty-four-hour duration of action, so a cup of coffee consumed at seven in the morning is still in your bloodstream at ten at night when you are trying to fall asleep. To avoid caffeine withdrawal, please taper off caffeine over several weeks.

Absolutely avoid alcohol within six hours of bedtime while going through insomnia treatment. For patients not suffering from insomnia, the recommendation is to avoid alcohol within three hours of bedtime.

Do not take over-the-counter sleeping pills without consulting your doctor. An ideal sleeping pill is one that gives you six to eight hours of sleep with a normal percentage of deep sleep without causing daytime grogginess. It is also important that any sleeping pill you choose does not lose effectiveness with time and does not lead to dependence. Your physician can help you decide the right medication at the right dosage. Remember, you should not take a sleeping pill without knowing the cause of your insomnia. And when you do take a sleeping pill, take it at the lowest possible dosage for the shortest duration.

If you are interested in herbal supplements, please read about chamomile tea, valerian root, and melatonin. You can visit the website of the National Center for Complementary and Alternative Medicine (NCCAM) at http://nccam.nih.gov for the current and credible information.

Chamomile is commonly used as a bedtime tea, but scientific evidence of its effectiveness for insomnia is lacking. The herb kava has been used for insomnia, but there is no evidence of its efficacy. The Food and Drug Administration (FDA) has issued a warning that kava supplements have been linked to a risk of severe liver damage.

Valerian is one of the most popular herbal therapies for insomnia, anxiety, depression, and menopause symptoms. Several studies suggest that valerian can improve the quality of sleep and slightly reduce the time it takes to fall asleep. However, not all the evidence is positive. One systematic review of the research concluded that, although valerian is commonly used as a sleep aid, the scientific evidence does not support its efficacy for insomnia.

Researchers have concluded that valerian appears to be safe at recommended doses for short-term use. No information is available about the long-term safety of valerian or its safety in children younger than age three, pregnant women, or nursing mothers. Side effects include headache, dizziness, itching, and digestive disturbances. Because it is possible (though not proven) that valerian might have a sleep-inducing effect, it should not be taken along with alcohol or sedatives.

Some sleep-formula products combine valerian with other herbs, such as hops, lavender, lemon balm, and skullcap. Although many of these other herbs have sedative properties, there is no reliable evidence that they improve insomnia or that combination products are more effective than valerian alone. Remember that the FDA has not tested the efficacy and safety of these supplements. Discuss these with your doctor.

Melatonin is a natural hormone that helps you fall asleep. Melatonin production and release in the brain is related to time of day, rising in the evening and falling in the morning. Light at night blocks its production. Melatonin dietary supplements have been studied for sleep disorders, such as jet lag, disruptions of the body's internal "clock," insomnia, and problems with sleep among people who work night shifts. It has also been studied for dementia symptoms.

Study results are mixed on whether melatonin is effective for insomnia in adults, but some studies suggest it may slightly reduce the time it takes to fall asleep.

Melatonin appears to be safe when used short-term, but the lack of long-term studies means we don't know if it is safe for extended use.

In one study, researchers noted that melatonin supplements may worsen mood in people with dementia. Side effects of melatonin are uncommon but can include drowsiness, headache, dizziness, or nausea.

Tell all your health care providers about any complementary or integrative health approaches you use. Give them a full picture of what you do to manage your health. This will help ensure coordinated and safe care.

Recognize that aromatherapy, using essential oils from herbs such as lavender or chamomile, is a popular sleep aid. Preliminary research suggests some sleep-inducing effects, but more studies are needed.

Music therapy can help too. Listening to relaxing music of your choice at bedtime can help, too. YouTube.com has a ten-minute music video by Dr. Jeffrey Thompson with more than eight million hits and great reviews from people suffering from insomnia. (You can check it out by searching "Jeffrey Thompson" on YouTube.com.)

Learn progressive muscle relaxation as discussed earlier. This is especially important if anxiety is contributing to your insomnia, because muscle relaxation is incompatible with anxiety. You can also try total relaxation, demonstrated in a ten-minute video on YouTube.com posted by Nancy Parker (coolkarmavideo is her YouTube.com user name). I find progressive muscle relaxation especially helpful when I cannot fall asleep after receiving a call from the hospital at night. You can try it when you cannot fall asleep after a trip to the restroom at night.

Learn mindfulness meditation. You can learn the technique on www.shambhalasun.com. You can also search for instructional videos on YouTube.com that teach to meditation techniques. A six-minute guided instructional video by Jim Malloy (jmalloy108) is extremely helpful.

Sleeping for Two? Try These Tips!

According to the National Sleep Foundation's 1998 women and sleep poll, 78 percent of women report more disturbed sleep during pregnancy than at other times. As we discussed earlier, sleep apnea is more common in pregnant females. It is vital that you sleep with CPAP to avoid fetal and maternal complications.

The following tips can help you sleep better.

1. Plan, schedule, and prioritize sleep. Follow sleep hygiene with twice the fervor and fanaticism as you are indeed sleeping for two.
2. Avoid caffeine completely because it will compound the problem of insufficient deep sleep. It being a diuretic will also make your frequency of urination worse.
3. After checking with your physician, exercise for at least thirty minutes per day.
4. Sleep on your left side to improve the flow of blood and nutrients to your fetus and your uterus and kidneys. Keep your knees and hips bent. Place pillows between your knees, under your abdomen, and behind your back. This may take pressure off your lower back. Try to avoid lying on your back for extended periods of time. You may try special pregnancy pillows, which can help you be comfortable during sleep.
5. Drink lots of fluids during the day, especially water, but cut down on the amount you drink in the hours before bedtime.
6. If you can't sleep for twenty minutes, don't lie in bed and force yourself to sleep. Get out of the bedroom, and read a relaxing book, knit or crochet something for your baby, write in a journal, or take a warm bath.

7. Learn progressive muscle relaxation. This will help your insomnia, and it will come in handy during delivery.

8. Avoid looking at bright light at night. A nightlight in the bathroom will be less stimulating, so it will allow you to return to sleep more quickly.

9. During work days, take a PREM power nap in the early afternoon. During weekends, you can take a longer nap in the afternoon to pay up your sleep debt. If you have difficulty falling asleep at night, then nap earlier in the day or curtail the duration of the nap.

10. In order to avoid heartburn, do not eat large amounts of spicy, acidic, or fried foods. Also, eat frequent small meals throughout the day.

11. Recognize that snoring is very common during pregnancy, but, if you have pauses in breathing, you should be screened for sleep apnea.

12. If you develop Restless Leg Syndrome, seek medical attention. Your doctor will check you for iron or folate deficiency. Keep your legs elevated at work and at home as much as you can. This can prevent leg swelling and may help your RLS. Leg stretching exercises can help RLS, too.

God bless you both!

Using CPAP during Menstruation

According to the National Sleep Foundation's Women and Sleep poll, half of menstruating women complain of disrupted sleep for three days each menstrual cycle even in the absence of sleep apnea. Using CPAP during menstruation poses an additional challenge. For females suffering from premenstrual syndrome, sleep disruption and the resultant drop in daytime alertness are even worse. Also, progesterone hormone, which peaks in the second half of the menstrual cycle, exacerbates fatigue and excessive daytime sleepiness. These recurring challenges can take a toll every month on these hardworking females.

The following tips can help. Remember that, if you master these interventions, you can use CPAP, spend more time in deeper stages of sleep and get recurring return on your investment month after month throughout your career.

1. Follow sleep hygiene with a fervor. Mother Nature is not helping you, so you will have to help yourself. Maintain regular sleep-wake schedule, avoid alcohol within 6 hours of bedtime, keep work related material out of bedroom, and keep your bedroom cool, quiet, and dark.

2. Remember that exercise will help you fight PMS symptoms and improve your REM sleep too.

3. Gradually taper caffeine off completely. Besides disrupting your deep sleep, caffeine contributes to premenstrual bloating.

4. Drink more during the daytime. Drink plenty of fluid all day, but stop drinking in the evening to avoid nocturnal urination.

5. Avoid the it-is-just-PMS attitude. Take your PMS seriously, and consult your physician to reduce PMS symptoms of bloating, breast tenderness, back pain, cramping, irritability, nervousness, and grumpiness.

6. Schedule lightly. You may argue that this is not always possible, but, with proper planning, you might be able achieve this. Try to squeeze in a PREM (Patel's REM) nap in your busy schedule if you can.

7. Do not let pride prevent you from seeking support. You know you are fighting Mother Nature, but no one else does because you cannot share this with your male

colleagues. But this should not prevent you from seeking support from your female colleagues and, for sure, your family members.

8. Learn progressive muscle relaxation and mindful meditation. This will help you deal with untoward emotions. It will also treat that feeling of powerlessness that you as a leader hate. To learn mindful meditation, you can watch this simple and useful video by Jim Malloy of http://www.meditationcenter.com.

9. Talk to your doctor about sleeping pills for occasional as needed use.

Sleep Soundly During Menopause

Obstructive sleep apnea is more common in males than in females, but at menopause, this difference narrows as the hormonal changes in females make their upper airway more collapsible. We do see quite a few postmenopausal females for sleep apnea, and insomnia mainly from hot flashes, joint pains, depression, or adverse effects from the medications. This insomnia makes it difficult for them to get used to CPAP.

During the transition phase leading to menopause, over several years, a woman's ovaries gradually decrease production of estrogen and progesterone. One year after menstrual periods have stopped, a woman reaches menopause, usually around the age of fifty. Menopause is a time of major hormonal, physical, and psychological change. Natural changes in sleep also occur, characterized by longer time to sleep onset, frequent awakenings, decreased amount of deep sleep, and poor sleep architecture.

From perimenopause to post menopause, women report

hot flashes, mood disorders, insomnia, and sleep-disordered breathing. Sleep problems are often accompanied by depression and anxiety, which make insomnia worse. This is the reason post-menopausal women are not satisfied with their sleep. As many as 61 percent report insomnia symptoms. Snoring and sleep apnea have also been found to be more common and more severe in post-menopausal women as their upper airway dilator muscles become flabby with aging.

Changing and decreasing levels of estrogen cause many menopausal symptoms, including hot flashes, which are unexpected feelings of heat all over the body accompanied by sweating. They usually begin around the face and spread to the chest, affecting 75 to 85 percent of women around menopause. On average, hot flashes last three minutes and lead to reduced sleep efficiency. Most women experience these for one year, but about 25 percent have hot flashes for five years. Hot flashes interrupt sleep and reduce the amount of deep sleep, leading to suboptimal alertness and suboptimal leadership the following day.

Talk to your doctor about estrogen (estrogen replacement therapy or ERT) or estrogen and progesterone (hormone replacement therapy or HRT), nutritional products, and medications such as calcium supplements, vitamin D, and bisphosphonates for the prevention or treatment of osteoporosis (thinning and weakening of the bones). Also, talk about estrogen creams and rings for vaginal dryness.

Discuss alternative treatment for menopausal symptoms such as soy products (tofu, soybeans, and soy milk). They contain phytoestrogen, a plant hormone similar to estrogen. Soy products may lessen hot flashes. Phytoestrogen is also available in over-the-counter nutritional supplements (ginseng, extract of red clover, or black cohosh). The FDA does not regulate these supplements. Their proper doses, safety, and long-term effects and risks are not yet known.

The following tips will help you sleep better with CPAP even during   menopause.

1. Avoid foods that are spicy or acidic because these may trigger hot flashes.

2. Try foods rich in soy because they might minimize hot flashes.

3. Avoid nicotine, caffeine, and alcohol, especially before bedtime. These will make your hot flashes worse.

4. Dress in lightweight clothes to improve sleep efficiency. Avoid heavy, insulating blankets, and consider using a fan or air-conditioner to cool the air and increase circulation. If your spouse is shivering, have a small, portable heater next to his side of the bed. You can also investigate the beds with dual temperature controls.

5. Reduce stress and worry as much as possible. Try relaxation techniques, massage, and exercise. Talk to a behavioral health professional if you are depressed, anxious, or having problems.

6. It is vital that you follow sleep hygiene instructions.

7. Try consolidating your sleep by going to bed thirty minutes later than your usual bedtime. As we age, we spend more time in bed, but we sleep less.

8. If you still have difficulty sleeping, talk to us about a sleep-aid.

Enjoy the Life Beyond Fifties!

Too Busy to Sleep Seven Hours?

There are times in our lives when we cannot get seven hours of sleep: a wedding in the family, an illness of a loved one, changes at work, and the likes. How can you be at your best despite insufficient sleep? What if this demand continues for days or weeks?

As the sleep debt increases, so does sleepiness. I used to be grumpy, irritable, achy, and sluggish after a busy night at the hospital. In the following pages, I will give you practical tips to help you maximize your alertness and improve your mood even when sleep-deprived. I have successfully tried them during my post-call days in the Intensive Care Unit for twenty years.

You can't improve what you can't measure. Monitor your alertness using Patel's Alertness Sleepiness Scale (PASS). For consistent excellence, you need to be at a ten all day long. Be aware of subnormal PASS at all times.

Patel's Alertness Sleepiness Scale (PASS)	
Feeling active, vital, alert, or wide awake	10
Functioning at high levels, but not at peak Able to concentrate	8
Awake, but relaxed Responsive but not fully alert	6
Somewhat foggy Let down	4
Foggy Losing interest in remaining awake Slowed down	2
Sleepy, woozy, fighting sleep Prefer to lie down	0

LAMP (Leader's Alertness Maximization Plan)

All day, and certainly during critical moments, measure and monitor your alertness using PASS. The surest and most natural cure for a low PASS is sleep, but what do you do when you cannot get sufficient sleep because of a hectic schedule and unavoidable demands? You can use the LAMP (Leader's Alertness Maximization Plan) to regain your alertness and thereby your life. Going against the might of Mother Nature, you can summon the help of these seven friends as applicable to your situation:

1. Physical exertion

2. PREM nap

3. Bright light

4. Caffeine

5. Smart snacking

6. Massage

7. Faith (my all-time favorite)

Also, beware of the formidable foe in alcohol when faced with insufficient sleep and long days.

• Keep moving. Get into the habit of standing at work. Walk,

walk, walk.

- Bright light has tremendous alerting influence. Use this to your advantage. Sit facing the window. During long meetings in the boardroom, look up at light often. Especially on cloudy days, put a bright light lamp behind your desktop while working on it. Every fifteen minutes, turn off the PowerPoint presentation and turn on the lights.

- Small protein snacks every two to three hours will maintain your energy and alertness while eating a large starchy meal will degrade your alertness. Grilled fish or chicken is fine. Avoid rice, pasta, and dessert.

- Caffeine has alerting property, but it has the duration of action of twenty-four hours, so a cup of coffee consumed at one o'clock is still in your bloodstream at midnight when your brain is trying to get into REM sleep. Because of this reason, caffeine should not be used indiscriminately. It should be used as a medicine, at the right dosage, at the right time, and for the right reason. The surest indication for caffeine is driving when sleep deprived. This can be lifesaving.

- A PREM (Patel's REM) nap can improve alertness for three hours. Studies have shown that a fifteen-minute nap can improve alertness and last for almost three hours.

- Massage especially when combined with a PREM nap can improve alertness because it relieves muscle aches, back pain, headaches, burning in the eyes, and other distracting physical symptoms precipitated by sleep deprivation. Untreated, these symptoms can drag your energy level and your alertness down.

- Spiritual support has helped me the most during my post-call days in the clinic. Going from one exam room to next, I would look up and ask for divine help. "Give me energy, my Lord, to serve my patients well."

Even the legal limit of alcohol will impair your leadership when sleep deprived. Avoid even a small glass of wine or a beer when sleep deprived. Resist that temptation.

Grumpy When Sleepy

The following list summarizes the deleterious effects of poor sleep on our emotional intelligence:

1. When sleep deprived, we are unable to accurately recognize emotions. To make matter worse, negative emotions are more readily recognized than positive ones.
2. Studies have shown decreased subjective rating of happiness by sleep-deprived people.
3. Our overactive fear center (Amygdala) exaggerates our fear and anger when sleep deprived.
4. Sleep deprivation impairs our social interaction and learning because of perception fatigue.
5. A study from the Neuroscience Lab in Singapore showed that when sleep deprived, we are reactive and not proactive.
6. Nervousness, irritability, and grumpiness hurt our teamwork.
7. Impaired self-evaluation resulting from sleep deprivation makes us unaware of our deficits.
8. Studies have also shown reduced motivation, increased risk taking, and indecisiveness when faced with an ethical dilemma.

Survival Tips When Tired

Even my most CPAP-compliant patients suffer from insufficient sleep when going through a challenge at work or at home. Some of them become grumpy, ill-tempered, and nervous running on too little sleep. This happens because of overstimulated Amygdala (our brain's fear center) and under-active Executive Center (Prefrontal Cortex of our brain). Here are a few tips I found immensely helpful during my post call days in the clinic and in the hospital.

1. Walk with a bounce and exude contagious enthusiasm and optimism.
2. Smile often. Recognize that smile is your savior. Stay close to people with positive demeanor. Humor and happiness stabilize our intellect.

3. Pause before answering. Save emotional e-mails in the drafts folder and send them the next morning. If it is a complicated issue or a vital one, sleep on it. Recognize that the pause is your partner.

4. Do not dwell on the unpleasant aspect of your work or of your   life.

5. Pray often. When on the go, read a line from Bible. Replace fear and anger with faith and empathy through mental discipline.

6. Take a walk, talk to your spouse, nap, meditate, exercise, and play. Beware of delicate situations that can exaggerate the irritability. Tactfully avoid them or live through them quietly.

Hence, make sure you get 7-8 hours of sound sleep every night with CPAP on. And when you cannot get sound sleep because of unavoidable factors, please beware of these deleterious effects. Smile often, pause before responding, listen more than you talk, and you will be fine.

Enjoy Peak Alertness Every Moment
Rectangular Alertness - Top of Your Game All-Day!

Even after following sleep hygiene with fervor, we feel sleepiness during mid-afternoon because of our internal clock. Some of feel sluggish in the morning as we are born as evening person, while others feel sluggish in the evening. How can we fight this? How can we regain these parts of our days such that we feel maximally alert all-day long? This is called rectangular alertness. When we achieve this, we get more out of our days. We reduce accidents and poor decisions.

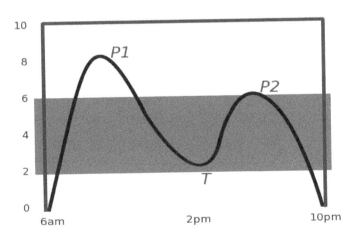

In the above graph, P1 and P2 refer to the peak alertness experienced by us in a typical day, while T refers to the trough in our alertness felt around mid-afternoon. By using the techniques discussed in this chapter, we can achieve the rectangular alertness and feel maximally alert all day long.

What are the benefits of the rectangular alertness? They are many, from the individual level to the national level:

☐ It can eliminate disastrous decisions and maximize executive output, both qualitatively and quantitatively.

☐ It can turn a good team into a high-performing team by eliminating suboptimal alertness and suboptimal performance during team meetings and beyond.

☐ It can ensure safety, quality, and optimum output by ensuring an alert workforce.

☐ Rectangular alertness can give the nation competitive advantage by having leaders and workers who are maximally alert all day long, even during a major catastrophe or a huge opportunity.

Live Your Life from the Highest Level of Wakefulness.

How to Become a Morning Person

My patients who consider themselves to be evening persons find it difficult to get started in the mornings. As a result, they end up missing out on 10 percent to 20 percent of the day and, in fact, of life, not to mention the potential for disastrous leadership while running early morning meetings.

Here, are a few tips that can help you become a morning person:

- Buy an alarm clock that simulates the sun rise. You can find one made by Phillips on Amazon. This has changed my life. I do not dread seeing patient at seven AM!
- As soon as your alarm goes off, get out of bed. Do not think. If you start thinking, you have lost the battle. Just get out of bed.
- Go from bed to bike and start pedaling. It can be immensely energizing. You can put your laptop on the stand and check your e-mails and plan your day as you are pedaling.
- If you are a coffee person, enjoy a flavorful cup of coffee. You can set the coffee pot on a timer to start brewing fifteen minutes before your alarm goes off.
- A hot shower can awaken you, too. Make sure you get out of the shower quickly.
- Bright light in the morning can be extremely helpful. Phillips makes an alarm clock that simulates sunrise. It works especially well on those dark winter mornings.

Eliminate the MADness (Mid Afternoon Drowsiness)

"I feel much more alert and energetic on CPAP, but I do still feel a little sleepy around 1 - 2 PM every day," a sixty year old office manager shared with me. Well, you are not alone. The majority of mammalian species have a second sleep period during the daytime because of this mid-afternoon dip in alertness. This dip in the alertness in the middle of our working day causes a decline in our productivity and, more importantly, creates an environment

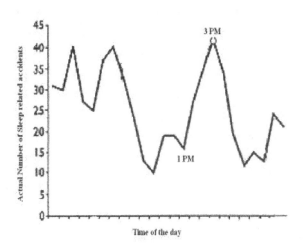

conducive to disastrous mistakes, and worse, fatal accidents.

The incidence of sleep-related vehicle accidents (n=606) by hour of day. BMJ 1995; 310: 565 Sleep-related vehicle accidents. JA Horne, professor, LA Reyner, research associate, Sleep Research Laboratory, Department of Human Sciences, Loughborough University, Leicestershire LE11 3TU.

Why does this occur? Well, our internal pacemaker, Suprachiasmatic nucleus located at the base of the brain makes us sleepy in the mid-afternoon. Fighting this tiny structure will take discipline and persistence, but this can improve your executive output by thirty percent and can eliminate disastrous decision making.

First, you have to recognize this decline in alertness and in productivity. Look for it and you shall find complacency and chaos, disastrous decision-making, and combustible communication post-lunch.

Keep these tips in mind to help you get through the mid-afternoon madness:

Keep moving. Pace the floor. If you are in a meeting, flex and extend your ankles. Take a trip to the restroom.

Look at the light. Sit facing the sun. Minimize power point use if giving a presentation. Turn the slides off and turn the lights on every ten minutes.

Eat a light lunch. If you avoid carbohydrates, you will not feel sluggish at the next afternoon meeting. Your head will be able to think clearly and handle crucial decision making duties.

Use caffeine judiciously. It can improve your alertness but can rob you of your deep sleep at night as it has duration of action of 24 hours.

Take a fifteen-minute power nap. It will go a long way in improving your performance as a leader. Studies have shown that a fifteen-minute power nap can improve alertness, decision-making, creativity, communication, perception, situational awareness, and problem-solving for 150 minutes. There are times I do not have time for the nap. During those times, closing eyes even for a couple of minutes help me stay alert and focused.

If you follow these tips, you can maximize alertness even in the afternoon.

Regain Your Evenings

Early-morning people run out of energy and end up underperforming in the evening meetings.

Here, are some tips you can use to regain your evenings:

☐ Plan and take a ten-to-fifteen minute PREM nap prior to three o'clock. This will give you a second wind in the evening.

☐ Avoid heavy meals in the evening.

☐ An evening walk or exercise can be alerting. Get up and start walking as soon as you notice lethargy creeping in.

☐ It breaks my heart to tell you that even a glass of wine can drag your alertness down. Resist that temptation, especially if you have an important event in the evening.

☐ Caffeine can be alerting, but it will rob you of your deep sleep. It is best to avoid it.

If you follow above recommendations, you can achieve the rectangular alertness.

An Alert, Energetic, & Enjoyable Monday

Have you noticed how sleepy, tired, lethargic, and complacent you feel on Mondays? My patients, even on CPAP, are not immune to this malady. Medical studies indeed have shown reduced productivity and increased errors on Mondays secondary to disrupted sleep schedule on weekends.

You can enjoy and excel at work even on Mondays by following LAMP. Try it and you shall change your Mondays for better.

Power Nap: a Sign of Wisdom, not Weakness

You have had a very busy week. You got barely five hours of sleep last night. You did use your CPAP though. Your day started at five in the morning. The schedule is tiring, even for a seasoned warrior like you. Opportunities are tremendous. Adrenaline is pumping. With meeting after meeting, phone call after phone call, and a hurried social lunch, it's two o'clock before you know it. And the board meets in an hour. You are expected to make a compelling case for a drastic change in the strategic direction that the company urgently needs. Your eyelids feel heavy. Neck muscles are tight. Information you have so painstakingly compiled does not look as clear as it did last night.

Can you present data clearly? Can you make your case passionately? Can you listen to their comments carefully? Can you gauge their mood? Can you perceive their interests accurately? Can you read between the lines? Can you separate people from the problem? Can you find common ground? Can you rally your colleagues for greater good? After a power nap, you certainly can!

Seven Strong Reasons to Take a Power Nap

Studies prove that a fifteen-minute power nap provides

benefits lasting up to 150 minutes, including:

1. Improved alertness, both subjectively and objectively
2. Reduced fatigue and improved vigor
3. Enhanced creativity and problem solving
4. Improved perception
5. Facilitated learning
6. Improved declarative and procedural memory
7. Positive mood and emotions, clearer communication, humor and optimism, and situational awareness

If a fifteen-minute nap gives you 150 minutes of improved function and health, how can you resist such an investment.

But how do you take this power nap? Relax. It's easy. You don't have to do anything hard. Of course, there is a definite learning curve, but you will get better as you take these power naps on a regular basis.

In research studies, participants were asked to take naps in a quiet, dark, and comfortable environment. You may not have such an environment at work, but with practice, you can still take a very invigorating and rewarding nap. Legend has it that a ferocious Mughal warrior, Aurangzeb, took naps while still sitting on his horse in the middle of the battlefield.

The biggest obstacle to the practice of power napping is the stigma it carries in our frenzied corporate culture, which looks at napping as a sign of weakness, not wisdom. How do you take a power nap then? As with most changes, this one also begins in your mind. Review the reasons for power naps and the benefits they offer. Analyze the data and make a rational decision. Next, share your plan to invest in power naps with people around you, starting with your spouse, your secretary, your closest colleague, and so on.

As appropriate, educate your staff and colleagues about the performance benefits of power naps. Inform them that napping is a sign of wisdom, not weakness. This will help you overcome that cultural barrier and stigma associated with daytime napping. Then show the confidence of a leader and just do it. It is not that difficult; and it is worth the trouble and time.

Most patients on CPAP do not need a power nap unless they are unable to get the necessary seven hours of sleep because of personal or professional reasons. But there are medical and practical reasons to err on the side of taking one. A nap in the afternoon can give you two days in one, as Churchill used to say. It does not have to be a long one like Churchill used to take. You do not even have to fall asleep during the nap. A ten minute shut-eye is all I need to keep on going at the clinic.

While talking to Dan Rather of CBS News in 1993, Bill Clinton said, "If I can take a nap—even fifteen or twenty minutes—in the middle of the day, it is really invigorating to me. On the days when I'm a little short of sleep, I try to work it out so that I can sneak off and just lie down for fifteen minutes, a half hour, and it really makes all the difference in the world."

Because of our internal circadian rhythm, our alertness and, hence, our performance dips in the afternoon. This nadir is deeper when we are sleep deprived and when we are traveling across multiple time zones. If we can fight this drowsiness with a strategically placed power nap, then we can maximize our efficiency and avoid fatal mistakes. (Most fatal vehicular accidents occur in the mid-afternoon and after midnight.)

Technique of a Conventional Power Nap

You want to learn how to nap? Well, do nothing and you shall be napping!

Following tips will you help you rejuvenate your day with a 15 minute power nap.

• Proudly let your staff know that you will be taking a fifteen-minute nap. "Doctor's orders," you may add.
• Set your Smartphone alarm, preferably on vibrate, to go off in fifteen minutes. A study from Australia has shown that napping for less than ten minutes is suboptimal. More than twenty minutes can be counterproductive because of post-nap grogginess.
• Turn on relaxing music. You can try noise-canceling headphones. Bose are the best.
• Put on eye shades. I find my Notre Dame cap very useful, especially when taking a nap in the public place. I just pull it down over my eyes, and I am off to the land of dreams.
• Stretch on the couch or recline in the chair. Turn the chair away from people and toward the window or wall. A study from China showed greater benefit with stretching on the couch as opposed to sitting.
• Close your eyes, shut off your mind, and relax.
• Wake up with a smile and vigor when the alarm goes off.

A Nap Improves Creative Problem-solving

A nap improves creative problem solving by a whopping 40 percent. An interesting study done by Dr. Sara Mednik and her team at University of California, San Diego, looked at creative problem solving before and after a nap. Participants were given three words and asked to find a word that can link all of the three words, for example, sixteen, candy, and heart. The answer is sweet: sweet sixteen, sweet candy, and sweet heart. There was an amazing 40 percent improvement after a nap containing REM sleep. (By the way, if you plan on taking a nap longer than twenty minutes, you must wear your CPAP as you are more likely to reach REM sleep during which your apnea is severe.)

Remember that REM sleep has an active brain in a paralyzed body. Mother Nature made it so we do not act out our dreams. Also, studies have shown that REM sleep has a tremendous amount of random, bizarre, and seemingly unrelated activity going on, which our brain is trying to connect together to make some sense of it. Some researchers believe this is why REM nap is able to boost creative problem solving by linking these random and totally unrelated activities together. This is the wildest and craziest form of thinking outside the box. Studies have shown that REM sleep plays a pivotal role in memory consolidation, too.

Can we do better than just lie down and relax for fifteen minutes? Can we modify our technique to make our nap more restorative, more recuperative, and more energizing? I think we can by adding just a few steps to our conventional nap. I should clarify that these recommendations are not based on any specific scientific studies, but my experience as a practicing sleep specialist and lifelong nap-taker.

Let us learn to take PREM (Patel's Relaxed Eye Muscles) nap.

- Read a couple of lines from the Bible, Gita or any other religious book before the nap. You can store them on your Smartphone and read them before setting up the fifteen-minute alarm. REM sleep, the sleep stage with vivid dreams, unfortunately, has predominantly negative emotions like fear, anxiety, guilt, and anger. Here, we are trying to replace them with joy, optimism, love, and faith.

Matthew 18:23–26, says, "Have faith in God. I assure you: If anyone says to this mountain, 'Be lifted up and thrown into the sea,' and does not doubt in his heart, but believes that what he says will happen, it will be done for him.

Luke 6:27–36 says, "But I say to you who listen: Love your enemies, do good to those who hate you, bless those who curse you, pray for those who mistreat you. If anyone hits you on the cheek, offer the other also."

Lord Krsna in Gita, "Give all your worries to me and work with patience and enthusiasm."

• Begin your nap with five to ten slow, deep, and regular breaths. Relax your whole body as you exhale. Control of breathing is control of life. Breathing, unlike heart rate, blood pressure, temperature, and gastrointestinal motility/secretions, is the only vital function that we can easily control. And it is a time-tested tool used for centuries to achieve relaxation.

• Progressive muscle relaxation is incompatible with somatic anxiety. So, by focusing on respiration and relaxation, we are getting rid of anxiety, both from our conscious and our subconscious. As you breathe in and out, relax the muscles of your eyeballs and then continue to relax all the other muscles from head to toe and drift down into a state of pleasant relaxation. Stay in this state of weightlessness. And when the alarm goes off, wake up with tremendous positive energy.

I call this my PREM nap! This revolutionary power nap taps

into REM sleep's restorative power and limitless creativity.

Please watch this seven minute instructional video and start regaining your afternoons and evenings.

https://youtu.be/lX4esi-3xzU

Happy Napping!

Meditate? Nap? You Decide!

All my life, I have taken naps to fight off those deadly afternoon lulls. I have encouraged my staff to do the same in the nap room at our clinic. The studies indeed have shown that a 15 minutes nap can give alertness lasting for about 165 minutes. Lately, though, I have been meditating instead for 15 minutes in the afternoon or evening and have been pleased with the energy and alertness provided by meditation.

Why does meditation provide more restoration that a nap? Well, the research by Dr. Richard Davidson (the University of Wisconsin) has shown that meditation results in the coherence of theta and beta waves. Such coherence improves the brain functioning, just like an orchestra coming together to play a symphony. This coherence does not occur during a nap since a 15-20-minute nap cannot reach the deep sleep (stage 3 or the delta sleep) even if you fall asleep.

Meditation, in addition, results in emotional and spiritual rejuvenation as you focus on the Divine and relax physically while focusing continually on your respirations.

During the meditation, you also accept your thoughts honestly and openly without passing a judgement. After this, you withdraw your attention into the Divine within. This process leads to emotional and cognitive rejuvenation, which does not happen with the nap.

Meditation improves my sleep at night, whereas a nap certainly longer than 20 minutes or alter than 3 PM can interfere with my night-time sleep.

Studies have also shown that a nap longer than 20 minute may be followed a period of grogginess, while post-meditation, there is no such danger.

But, the most important reason is this. When I tell my wife that I need an afternoon nap, I get a nod of disapproval, but when I tell her I am going to meditate for 20 minutes, I get an instant approval! In her mind, a nap is a sign of laziness (and not of wisdom), while meditation is a sign of the divine dedication.

In conclusion, if you know how to meditate, try it in the afternoon or evening. If you don't know how to meditate, learn it and use it. You will rejuvenate your afternoons and evenings! If you can't learn to meditate, go ahead and take a nap — doctor's order!

7 Things You Shouldn't Do When Sleepy!

There are times that even CPAP patients feel sleepy. Maybe you had a cold and did not get enough sleep. Maybe you are working long hours or odd hours. It will be very tempting to make a snap decision and get on with your day, but there are things you should not do when sleepy.

1. Make financial decisions. Insufficient sleep affects our judgement, our information management ability, and our risk taking adversely. Please pay up your sleep debt first before making those costly financial decisions.

2. Make career decisions. Insufficient sleep also impairs our creativity, our big picture skills, and our self-assessment ability. Take a lazy vacation with your spouse, catch up on your sleep, relax on the beach, read a spiritual book, and only

then make that major decision.

3. Initiate negotiations with a formidable adversary at work or at home. Sleep debt unfortunately impairs our communication, perception, humor appreciation, and our information management. It makes us a poor negotiator, hence resist that urge to walk into the corner office asking for a favor.

4. Fire back. When we receive an emotional e-mail while sleep deprived, we have an irresistible urge to fire back. Hold your horses. Take a deep breath. Smile. Type a reply, but save it in the draft folder. Sleep on it, edit it, and send it the next morning.

5. Drive. Every hour on US roads, 2 people die because of drowsy driving. If you must drive, take a PREM nap, have a cup of strong coffee, and then drive carefully.

We have discussed how you can live well and lead well even when sleep deprived. You can practice these interventions as it applies to your particular situation. For my post-call days in the clinic, I found the following Ten Commandments for the Sleep Deprived immensely helpful. I hope you do. In the next section, we will learn how to leverage maximal alertness to achieve consistent executive excellence and then how to maximize our God-given potential by incorporating the greed for greater good and spiritual fervor.

Ten Commandments for the Sleep Deprived

1. Thou shall never make important decisions while sleep deprived. If we all were completely honest, we would sometimes admit to making a decision when we were too sleepy to make sense of the situation. Never make an

important decision when you are sleepy.

2. Thou shall always speak slowly, softly, and clearly. Verbal fluency is adversely affected when we are sleepy. We tend to eat our words, rush our sentences, and confuse our colleagues. Take it easy. Slow down. Speak clearly.

3. Thou shall not get upset when the whole world does not yield to you. Sleep-deprived people have this odd way of thinking. They truly believe that the sun rises and sets at their whim. They truly believe that employees will jump through hoops and bend over backwards, and they are quick to get angry when that does not happen. See what a lack of sleep can do to you?

4. Thou shall stretch your body, gently massage your eyes, and take a timely PREM nap. If you find yourself falling asleep at your desk, take action. Stand up, stretch your body, and gently massage your eyes for a few seconds. Then sit back down in your chair, and take a quick nap. You will be surprised what only a few minutes can do for your body.

5. Thou shall strive for excellence in everything you do. When sleep deprived, we have a natural tendency to just finish the work and head home without thinking about the quality of our work. So remember, in order to become an effective leader, you must strive for excellence and lead well even when you are sleep deprived.

6. Thou shall be nice to yourself and reward yourself for excellent work. When sleep deprived, we have a tendency to be critical of ourselves. Fight that tendency and congratulate yourself for excelling despite sleep deprivation. Reward yourself with a glass of wine or a

relaxing massage at the end of the day.

7. Thou shall postpone appropriate work for a well-rested you later on. A great leader will not try to make decisions when too sleepy to think clearly. Presidents, heads of corporations, nonprofit executives, and others all have a history of saying, "Let me sleep on this." And guess what? It does work!

8. Thou shall look for humor, smile often, and even laugh out loud, especially when things get worse. If things are getting out of control and not working out the way you need them to, start looking at the brighter side. Smile, and try to enjoy the moment.

9. Thou shall always walk away from a complex problem, an argument, or a tough adversary. If you are too sleepy and find yourself in the middle of a complex problem that needs your immediate attention, find a way to walk away. There is no shame in saying that you need more time to make a crucial decision. A good leader knows the importance of walking away.

10. Thou shall never eat a heavy meal when sleep deprived. Have you ever been sleep deprived and then decided to eat a very heavy meal? Remember the outcome? It made your ability to make a sensible decision even worse, and, at the same time, it was damaging to your health. If you find yourself sleep deprived, instead of heading to the kitchen for a bite to eat, head to the nap room for some much-needed rest.

We learned how we can be maximally alert even when faced with unavoidable sleep deprivation. In the next section, we shall learn how we can leverage this alertness to improve emotional intelligence and informational intelligence. Add selflessness and spiritual power to this and you have the model for a supreme life.

Section V
Live a Supreme Life on CPAP

Inspirational Quotes for Business and Work Excellence

The secret of joy in work is contained in one word, excellence. To know how to do something well is to enjoy it. (Pearl Buck)

The quality of a person's life is in direct proportion to their commitment to excellence, regardless of their chosen field of endeavor. (Vince Lombardi)

Excellence, then, is not an act but a habit. (Aristotle)

Desire is the key to motivation, but it is determination and commitment to an unrelenting pursuit of your goal—a commitment to excellence—that will enable you to attain the success you seek. (Mario Andretti)

The companies that survive longest are the ones that work out what they uniquely can give to the world, not just growth or money but their excellence, their respect for others, or their ability to make people happy. Some call those things a soul. (Charles Handy)

The test of the artist does not lie in the will with which he goes to work, but in the excellence of the work he produces. (Thomas Aquinas)

Whatever your discipline, become a student of excellence in all things. Take every opportunity to observe people who manifest the qualities of mastery. These models of excellence will inspire you and guide you toward the fulfillment of your highest potential. (Michael Gelb and Tony Buzan)

You use CPAP religiously now. You follow sleep hygiene. You feel maximally alert all the time. Now, what? How can you use this alertness to squeeze out most life out of every moment? How can you use this alertness to be the best leader at work and at home? This is where the AEI model comes into play. It helps you manage your Alertness, Emotions, and Information to achieve consistent excellence. It further helps you cherish every moment this life gifts you. So, learn this model, use it daily, lead bravely, and live fully. Here, is an abridged version of this model. If interested, you can read more about this life-enhancing, and life-changing model in my first book, Sleep Well, Lead Well.

AEI Model of Consistent Excellence

Why is your performance great one day, average the next, and mediocre when the crisis strikes at home or at work? What makes your executive output inconsistent despite the same ability, same expertise, and same brain? Is it just a statistical phenomenon based on the laws of probability? Does the performance have to assume a bell-shaped curve? Can you always blame macroeconomic factors for such inconsistent performance? How about factors within an individual? Could suboptimal alertness and resultant drop in emotional intelligence and informational intelligence cause this?

Inconsistent alertness leads to inconsistent leadership, and suboptimal alertness leads to suboptimal leadership. Studies have shown that maximal alertness can lead to consistent excellence. But since it is not always possible to be maximally alert, how do you maximize your God-given potential despite suboptimal alertness?

How do you recognize and overcome task–ability mismatch when a major crisis hits? When you are low on your alertness scale, hence low on your emotional intelligence score and your informational intelligence scale, how can you still be the best leader you can be? This is where the AEI program comes to the rescue.

The goal of the AEI program is to maximize your God-given potential and achieve true excellence, as opposed to truncated, suboptimal, inconsistent, and, hence, pseudo-excellence.

Medical Evidence for AEImax Model

Our alertness fluctuates because of homeostatic drive (how long we have been awake) and our internal pacemaker, the suprachiasmatic nucleus, which makes us sleepy during mid-afternoon and at night. This decline is steeper and deeper in the presence of sleep deprivation.

The role of emotional intelligence in the leadership function has been well documented. What is overlooked, though, is the inconsistency in emotional intelligence, which contributes to the inconsistency in the executive function. A fluctuating level of alertness is the primary reason for emotional intelligence inconsistencies in the same leader at different times.

Numerous studies have also shown that, as alertness declines, so does information intelligence (ability to understand, process, store, apply, and reproduce information).

We can reach an AEImax state of leadership when we maximize our Alertness, then leverage that alertness to maximize our Emotional intelligence and Information intelligence. Once we successfully eliminate internal factors responsible for inconsistency and truncated excellence, we can capitalize on external factors, both organizational and global. This is the state of AEImax, when the leader is at the peak of executive excellence, firing on all cylinders.

When you achieve the state of AEImax by design and discipline, you, as a person and as a leader, are in the zone. This is when you should make vital decisions affecting your personal, professional, and family life.

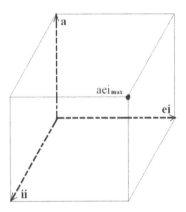

The above graph shows how one can, at a given moment, reach AEImax by maximizing alertness and then leveraging it to maximize EI and II.

Can you sustain this state of AEImax all day long? Can you be in the zone all the time? Remember, Mother Nature did not program our brain to be maximally alert sixteen hours a day every day. Also, today's global economy and executive expectations make it difficult to get eight hours of quality sleep every day of the year.

How can you be in the zone when the market crashes in Japan, volcanoes erupt in Iceland, or key financial institutions collapse? Or when a close family member gets admitted to ICU, your co-worker takes a week off unexpectedly during a hectic season, or a major catastrophic event strikes your family?

It is difficult, but not impossible. This long and rewarding journey toward being in the zone all the time starts with alertness intelligence, which begins with a fanatical discipline to follow sleep hygiene to maximize alertness. It also includes a continual and pleasant awareness of one's own and others' alertness, but most importantly, it involves learning and applying the countermeasures discussed in the Leader's Alertness Maximization Plan earlier. This will result in maximal alertness, which can last all day long.

Once you acquire rectangular alertness, you are ready to work on your emotional intelligence (self-awareness, self-management, motivation, interpersonal intelligence, social skills, and, most importantly, empathy). Developing unconditional empathy for your colleagues (especially those who do not agree with you), your customers (even those who complain about your product), your suppliers, and other stakeholders will help you become the best leader you can be. Follow the tips described in Section III to maintain empathy, optimism, enthusiasm, and social skills even when leading on insufficient sleep.

Next, you can work on your informational intelligence, which begins with an insatiable thirst for correct and useful information, along with the unique ability to receive, distill, digest, retain, apply, and reproduce it in an easy-to-understand manner. True leaders acquire almost a Zen-like ability to focus on relevant information and zone out unnecessary information. They continually develop and use this informational intelligence to become the most knowledgeable person in the industry and the best speaker in their organization. Having achieved maximal alertness, emotional intelligence, and informational intelligence, you can proudly say that you are an AEImax leader.

At all times, an AEImax leader is maximally alert, full of positive emotions, and the best informed and most knowledgeable person in the industry.

Ten Steps to AEImax

Reaching the AEImax state of leadership takes patience and perseverance. These recommendations will help you get started in the right direction:

1. Follow sleep hygiene with fervor. Guard your sleep like you guard your bottom line, because they are intricately tied together.
2. Develop alertness awareness. Throughout the day and at critical moments, use PASS (Patel's Alertness Sleepiness Scale) to rate your alertness.
3. With practice and persistence, eliminate preventable causes of sleep deprivation.
4. Expertly use countermeasures to neutralize midafternoon grogginess and jet-lag inefficiency.
5. Use PREM naps routinely to maximize your alertness and your leadership.
6. Continue to develop your emotional intelligence with a particular focus on empathy.
7. Be pleasantly aware of your emotional intelligence throughout the day, definitely during the critical moments.
8. Learn to manage information effectively with special focus on distilling information for greater good.
9. Be the most educated and informed person in the industry

by being a lifelong student. Remember that continuing education is infinitely more important than conventional education, as it is more relevant and more pertinent to the task at hand. By focusing on continuing education, dropouts such as Steve Jobs and Bill Gates excelled in their industry. Mahatma Gandhi rightly said, "Live as if you were to die tomorrow; learn as if you were to live forever."

10. Practice and improve your listening and public-speaking skills to be the best listener and speaker in the industry.

AEI∞ Model of a Supreme Life

You have trained your brain for consistent and sustainable leadership through AEImax. Do you use this newly acquired asset for personal pride, profit, and prestige, or do you use it for greater good? If you use AEImax for greater good, as opposed to personal profit, can it elevate your leadership and life to unimaginable heights? Do you let your core competency restrict your goal setting, or do you use your faith and spiritual power to push your abilities to new heights? Would you let macroeconomic malaise keep you down, or will your deep faith push you to persevere? This is where selflessness and spiritual strength come into play.

Mahatma Gandhi was not the smartest lawyer of his time; Bill Gates was far from being the smartest student in his class. But what they had was a very narrow and well-defined passion that they used for greater good and an unshakeable faith that allowed them to maximize their contribution to the human race by persevering year after year, through ups and downs in their long but rewarding journeys. The following is a graphic representation of how an AEImax leader can achieve such remarkable feats using selflessness and spiritual energy to become an AEI∞ leader.

Selfless service and spiritual power will catapult your leadership from AEImax to AEI∞.

The following graph gives a pictorial description of this helpful concept.

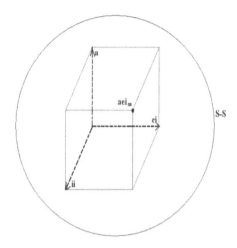

There is no salvation but through selfless service. Selfless service and greed for greater good will transform your leadership.

Two young monks had to cross the river and reach the temple before sunrise so they could attend the prayer meeting that the visiting guru was presiding over. Excited about this golden opportunity for a rare spiritual experience, they took off in the early morning hours, arrived at the river, got in the boat, and started rowing toward the temple. When the sky became dimly lit before the actual sunrise, they discovered to their surprise and shock that the boat was still anchored and had moved only the length of the rope. This is, unfortunately, the typical journey for most of us. Unless and until we untie ourselves from this self-centered anchor, we will not achieve our God-given potential.

Anne Morriss of Concire Leadership Institute has studied leaders around the world and shared her findings in the Harvard Business Review. She found consistently in each case that, at some point in their career, these leaders had undergone a remarkable transformation, when they started thinking, speaking, and acting for greater good, as opposed to personal profit, pride, and prestige.

Long Journey to the Promised Land

Unsure of his direction in the days before GPS navigation, a motorist pulls over, shows an address to a teenager, and asks, "How far is this place?" The young man looks at the address and the direction the motorist is heading. "Twenty thousand miles!" After a pregnant pause, he adds, "But if you turn around, it is only two miles. The road is uphill and a little bumpy initially, but it is a beautiful and scenic route. I am sure you would love it."

Most of us are on this twenty-thousand-mile journey to our destination. We think constantly about our interests, goals, prestige, and profits. We need to change this from the root level up, and begin thinking about our customers, colleagues, company, country, environment, and human race. And when we do that, only then will we maximize our God-given potential and contribute to the advancement of the human race to the best of our ability.

Selfless Action: A Darwinian Paradox?

The most difficult internal struggle we encounter as leaders is the struggle between self-centered thinking and selfless thinking. Our natural inclination for the former stems from the survival instinct ingrained in our genetic makeup. Our overstimulated amygdala compels us to act on this reptilian instinct, which must be annihilated with the fierce power of the executive center, the prefrontal cortex.

Two main factors can help a leader fight this survival

instinct: disciplined personal finances and a deep-rooted passion for the cause. Very few leaders can develop a passion reaching the depths acquired by Dr. King or Mahatma Gandhi; each man's passion made his survival instinct so obsolete that his fervor for his cause solely determined his actions. Developing a strong oneness with their cause can help leaders get started on this journey. Then persistence, passion, patience, and perseverance can help them become the selfless leaders they are capable of being.

You begin that journey internally, first by replacing self-centered thoughts one by one with externally directed thoughts. Have you noticed how industry leaders always think and talk about greater good? You can do that, too. Think of what is best for the department, company, industry, community, country, and human race. In doing so, you will grow as a global leader, you will be able to maximize your God-given potential, and you will reach AEI∞.

The 80/20 Rule of Selflessness

History is riddled with people who achieved greatness and served humanity, but ignored family responsibilities and ended up with a severely imbalanced life. Other leaders have maintained that delicate balance, and achieved the enormous feat of serving both their immediate families and the human race. You can successfully achieve this balance by following the 80/20 rule of selflessness. This rule recommends that you think, speak, and act for the greater good 80 percent of the time, and for yourself and your immediate family 20 percent of the time. You do not have to change your career. Just do the same work, but with an attitude of selfless service and you will achieve this feat. This rule will help you achieve AEI∞ without the imbalance that can cripple your life.

Spiritual Strength: An Underutilized Asset

If you say to this mountain, "Be lifted and thrown into the sea" and do not doubt, it shall be done for you.

"We Did Not Dream Big Enough"

The University of Notre Dame began on the bitterly cold afternoon of November 26, 1842, when a twenty-eight-year-old French priest, the Reverend Edward Sorin, and seven companions took possession of 524 snow-covered acres in the Indiana mission fields. In 1879, when a disastrous fire destroyed the main building, which housed virtually the entire university, Father Sorin vowed to rebuild the university and continue its growth.

"I came here as a young man and dreamed of building a great university in honor of Our Lady," he said. "But I built it too small, and she had to burn it to the ground to make the point. So, tomorrow, as soon as the bricks cool, we will rebuild it, bigger and better than ever."

That campus has grown from 524 acres in 1842 to 1,250 acres and 138 buildings in 2010. The University of Notre Dame today is a leading academic institution in the world. This would not have been possible without Father Sorin's unshakeable faith and deep spirituality.

Sleep deprivation adversely affects our faith and makes us ignore and, hence, underutilize our spiritual strength. We need to be cognizant of this handicap and find a routine such as prayer, regular meditation, frequent visits to our church, or continual consultation with our spiritual guru. Then we should stick to it, especially when setting our goals in life, planning our career, or facing adversity on our journey. Remember, faith sustains leadership.

Sleep deprivation's adverse effect on faith unfortunately gets worse with aging. Have you noticed how younger leaders demonstrate unbridled enthusiasm, set audacious goals, carry crazy creativity, and possess bold ideas? For most of us, aging, reality, and our work experiences moderate these qualities. Leaders, on the other hand, continue to nourish, nurture, and grow such enthusiasm and creativity throughout their long careers because of their deep faith. This unshakeable faith annihilates their amygdala's irrational fear and helps them reach their true potential.

The human race demands revolutionary ideas, actions, and results from its leaders. The only way a leader can deliver on this demand is by harnessing and utilizing spiritual strength. Deep faith and spiritual strength will help us see a future we can shape together for the advancement of the human race. Without faith and spiritual strength, Mahatma Gandhi could not have successfully sold his idea of nonviolence to three hundred million Indians, most of them illiterate, despite state-controlled media. When faced with insurmountable obstacles while working on our vision, a deep faith and spiritual strength will propel us past the problems.

Seven Steps to AEI∞ Leadership

How can we successfully get to the AEI∞ state of leadership? The following steps should help you get started on this long and rewarding journey:

Disciplined personal finances will help your journey toward

selflessness. Make an effort to keep in touch with those who practice simple living and high thinking. Frequently visit the website www.zenhabits.net, and moderate your urge to spend lavishly. Happiness does not come from owning, but from doing and giving. Self-indulgence that ties you up in a career you don't want is a noose around your neck. If you untie it and go for greater good, you will realize your God-given potential.

Frugal families can serve a greater good. Solicit your spouse's and children's cooperation in your quest for greater good. They are your closest allies and strongest supporters. You will be amazed at how much cooperation you get when you patiently discuss your passion and demonstrate self-restraint, discipline, and willpower. This may not happen overnight, but with love, faith, and persistence, you will receive the cooperation and support of your loved ones.

Look for common interests and actions that can help you personally and help your industry and your community. Slowly advance this process as you follow the 80/20 rule of selflessness. Think, speak, and act 80 percent of the time for the greater good and 20 percent of the time for your immediate family. This rule will help you achieve supreme leadership without ignoring your family. Learn to think, speak, and act as a global leader destined to leave a legacy for generations to come.

Humans learn best by observing. Mentor with a leader in the industry who has devoted his or her life selflessly to a noble cause. It might take patience, perseverance, and street smartness to find such a mentor, but you will be amazed by the number of true leaders who will find time in their busy schedules to teach their treasure of wisdom to a worthy devotee.

Make a conscious effort to encourage selflessness in your colleagues and family members. This will also help you in your own journey toward selflessness.

Choose a spiritual guru and keep in close contact. Attend a spiritual retreat every six months. Buddha said, "Be in the company of the wise, or better yet live with them."

Develop a daily prayer routine. Pray in the morning and at bedtime. With immovable faith, read one paragraph from the Bible or any other religious book three times a day. When you are extremely busy and on the go all the time, you may not have enough time for a complete prayer, but a line or two on the go will suffice. "Come, Holy Spirit" is what Father Theodore Hesburgh recites religiously when he wakes up, before he retires to bed, and several times during the day. Such practice will recharge your spiritual engine and allow you to tap into that unending source of energy.

Serve, Pray, and Lead

At all times, an AEI∞ leader is maximally alert, full of positive emotions, and the best informed and most knowledgeable person in the industry and in the family. And this leader is continually striving for greater good with unshakeable faith and deep spirituality.

In this book, I have tried to convince you to take your sleep seriously. Only through sound sleep, you can regain and recharge your life. Learn to achieve rectangular alertness. Leverage this alertness to maximize your emotional intelligence and your informational intelligence. Use it selflessly with spiritual strength to achieve soaring success.

Behavior change takes time, patience, and persistence. Follow me on twitter.com/yatinjpatel and receive my tweets about sleep disorders, sound sleep tips, sleep news, leadership, and life. Here are a few of my past tweets:

Pleasant and perpetual perception is a prerequisite to consistent excellence.

Sleep on your back and avoid facial wrinkles.

As I dream 2night, my Lord, take me to enchanted corners of every galaxy.

Dreams are a testament to brain's limitless imagination. Dream well 2night.

As I sleep, my Lord, replace hatred from my subconscious with faith and love. Good night 2 all.

Austerity of speech consists in speaking truthfully and beneficially & in avoiding offensive speech.

Imagination is a virtue of REM sleep more than of wakefulness.

REM sleep is the epicenter of innovation.

Teens need 9 hrs. sleep 2B happy, smart, & safe driver. It is 9 PM EST. Teens go 2 bed, Uncle Doc's order!

Awake, I am in Goshen. Asleep, I am everywhere.

Sleep is temporary death. And death is temporary sleep. Have a blast every moment.

We are what we think. Let us have noble thoughts today. Great morning to all!

Humor and happiness stabilize a leader's intellect.

Even when sleepy, spread contagious enthusiasm & optimism across the organization.

Do not dwell on unpleasant aspect of your work. REM sleep will magnify these negative emotions.

Be the most educated and informed person in the industry by being a lifelong student.

Accidents and poor decisions occur @ mid-afternoon. Drive alert. Sleep on a tough decision.

Wakefulness is the way to life.

Live a lifetime in each moment by pleasant and maximal alertness.

*As I sleep, Lord, fill up my vast subconscious with hope, happiness, joy, & bliss. And
then wake me up with highest level of consciousness.*

Kill Monday morning blues today. Walk with a bounce, talk with a smile, and work with joy.

Help me serve humanity with unshakable faith, empathy, and enthusiasm. Great morning to all.

Do not fight Mother Nature. Maintain regular sleep wake schedule this weekend and avoid Monday morning blues.

Truncated alertness leads to truncated life. Can infinite alertness lead to infinite life?

Post lunch dip in alertness leads to disastrous mistakes. Avoid heavy lunch today. Plan a power nap. Keep moving. Face the light.

Sleep is temporary death. Is death temporary sleep?

ABOUT THE AUTHOR

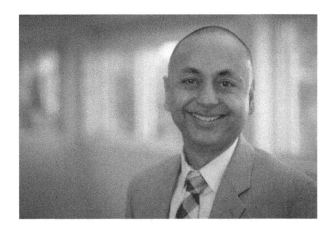

Hello!

I am a board certified pulmonary and sleep physician, a published author, and a passionate promoter of sleep and selfless leadership, currently enjoying my medical practice at Sneeze & Snooze Clinic, Goshen, Indiana.

With the help of my colleagues at Goshen Hospital, I founded the Center for Sleep Studies in 1994 and did the first sleep study in a small room, which was used for stress test during daytime! We have grown to a stand-alone, 4 bed sleep center accredited by American Academy of Sleep Medicine.

Son of a Gujarati writer publisher, I grew up in a small, dusty, hot village in Western India. After finishing my medical college in India, I immigrated to USA and started my internal medicine residency at Englewood Hospital in Englewood, NJ (a Mount Sinai Medical Center, New York's program). I served as the Chief Resident in the third year of the training program. After that, I finished pulmonary and sleep fellowship at Marshall University in Huntington, WV, and founded, in 1994, Sneeze & Snooze Clinic in Goshen, a beautiful little town in the middle of Amish country in Northern Indiana.

I am a senior fellow at American College of Chest Physicians and American Academy of Sleep Medicine, where I am also an active member of the Sleep Deprivation subcommittee.

Passionate about sleep, alertness, and driving safety, we started in 2002 our public awareness campaign, "Stay Awake, Drive Safe," aimed at eliminating drowsy driving-related accidents through educational events at schools, colleges,

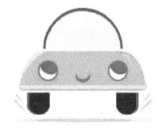

Stay Awake, Drive Safe

and highway rest plazas.

In 2008, I graduated magna cum laude from the Executive MBA Program, Mendoza College of Business, at the University of Notre Dame.
To educate the overworked executives on importance of sound sleep, and to help these sleep-deprived executives excel despite insufficient sleep, I wrote my first book - Sleep Well, Lead Well - which empowers them through a

transformational concept called, "The AEI∞ model of Supreme Leadership."

Perturbed by patients inability to afford life-saving treatment, we started in 2010, a non-profit initiative **CPAP for All** in partnership with Philips Respironics to help these patients receive CPAP treatment for free or at a nominal cost.

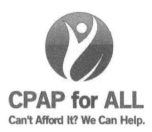

In 2012, I wrote my second book - Deeper Sleep, Richer Life - to help sleep-deprived females feel alert and energetic all-day, every day.

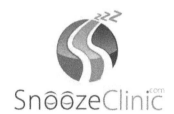

We started in 2014, an eStore http://SnoozeClinic.com with a mission that every patient with sleep apnea should get treated for under a $1000. On this eStore, we provide, along with intensive education through blogs and video clips, a few well-selected, quality products at the lowest price in the world.

I love public speaking, teaching, & media appearances. I blog, tweet, & talk @ sleep disorders, sound sleep tips, drowsy driving, success, women's rights & life.

Through our non-profit initiative called F.E.M.A.L.E. (Food, Education, Medications, And Love for Everyone) Ashram, my wife, Dipti, and I support the schools in the remote villages we both grew up in.

My hobbies include nature, meditation, philosophy, wine, and vegetarian cooking. I enjoy riding my bike on Pumpkin Vine Trail from Goshen to Shipshewana.

I live in Goshen, Indiana with my lovely wife, Dipti in our empty nest. Our three wonderful kids; two daughters Priyata and Pooja, and a son Parth left Goshen for the East Coast to pursue higher education.

It has been a remarkably rewarding journey helping thousands of patients, working with the area physicians, making lifelong friends locally, and watching our kids grow into smart, hard-working, compassionate, and responsible adults. I never forget my roots though. Here, is my picture wearing my grandpa's traditional hat and holding his stick outside our ancestral home in a small village in the western state of Gujarat in India!

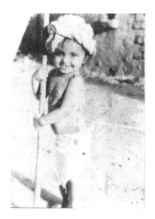

Sleep, Love, & Repeat.

Feel free to contact me at Doc@SnoozeClinic.com